"This is an excellent resource for MRCPsych students. It provides wide coverage of the curriculum while delivering the key details that make the difference in examinations."

Joanna Moncrieff, Reader in Critical and Social Psychiatry, Division of Psychiatry, UCL, UCL MRCPsych course organiser

"I have found the revision guide so helpful when preparing for the MRCPsych Part A exam. It is presented in an informative and concise manner and has been a great resource to use, especially when revising on the go. It was a great help towards passing the exam, I would highly recommend!"

Dr. Fraser MacNicoll, Core Trainee in Psychiatry

Revision Guide for MRCPsych Paper A

This text covers the key information necessary to pass Paper A of the postgraduate examination to become a member of the Royal College of Psychiatrists (MRCPsych). It emphasises memory aids in the forms of diagrams or tables, a novel presentation of these materials, providing a quick and portable source for pre-exam revision and visual memory aids and prompts.

Richard Kerslake, MBBS, MRCPsych, is a higher trainee in general adult and older persons psychiatry. He is a graduate of the Royal Free and University College London medical school. Dr. Kerslake is currently based in Sussex, England, having previously worked at Orygen Youth Health, Melbourne, and then completed core training in London. He is currently an honorary clinical lecturer at Brighton & Sussex Medical School where he has a special interest in simulation-based education and training of physician associates.

Elizabeth Templeton, MBChB, MRCPsych, trained at the University of Liverpool and graduated with honours in 2006. She moved to London soon after to start her psychiatric core training within the Camden and Islington Foundation Trust. Dr. Templeton has always had a keen interest in medical education; she has contributed to OSCEsmart, a published revision guide for practical exams, and she has played a significant role in the development of a pan-London simulation-based training programme. Dr. Templeton is now a specialist registrar in East London.

Lisanne Stock, BMBCh, MRCPsych, graduated from the University of Oxford and completed her foundation and core training in North Central London, where she continues to work as a higher trainee in general adult psychiatry. Dr. Stock has an interest in medical education and co-runs the CASC In Hand tailored revision course for the final part of the MRCPsych examinations. Dr. Stock is also a trustee for the charity Nip in the Bud, which aims to improve recognition of mental health conditions in primary school children via film.

Revision Guide for MRCPsych Paper A

Richard Kerslake
Elizabeth Templeton and
Lisanne Stock

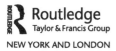

Routledge
Taylor & Francis Group

NEW YORK AND LONDON

First published 2018
by Routledge
711 Third Avenue, New York, NY 10017

and by Routledge
2 Park Square, Milton Park, Abingdon, Oxon, OX14 4RN

Routledge is an imprint of the Taylor & Francis Group, an informa business

ISBN: 978-0-815-36389-7 (hbk)
ISBN: 978-1-498-71613-0 (pbk)
ISBN: 978-1-315-11822-2 (ebk)

DOI: 10.1201/9781003322573

Typeset in Times New Roman
by Apex CoVantage, LLC

Contents

2   Basic and Social Psychology   15

ELIZABETH TEMPLETON

3 Sociocultural Psychiatry 32
ELIZABETH TEMPLETON

PART II
Human Development 43

4 Theories of Human Development 45
RICHARD KERSLAKE

PART III

Basic Neurosciences

5 Neuroanatomy

ELIZABETH TEMPLETON

6 Neurophysiology   **78**

ELIZABETH TEMPLETON

17 Psychopathology   181

RICHARD KERSLAKE

18 Diagnosis and ICD-10 Classification Codes 198

RICHARD KERSLAKE

Acknowledgements

Firstly, we would like to acknowledge our spouses, Taryn, Thomas and Alan. Without your support and the support of our families we wouldn't have been able to find the endless hours to study, collate and write the information that has been produced for this book.

Secondly, we would also like to thank Romayne Gadelrab who, with her unique combination of skills in graphic design and psychiatry, has produced the majority of illustrations for this book.

We would also like to thank Bhaskar Punukollu who has motivated us to reach the final stages of publication and who, with Abigail Swerdlow, was instrumental in the early stages of planning to bring this book into existence.

Thanks also to Michael Phelan and Anish Unadkat for their support and authoring of the preceding title, *MRCPsych in a Box*.

Introduction

*Richard Kerslake, Elizabeth Templeton
and Lisanne Stock*

This book was conceived after we have finished our written MRCPsych exams. We believed that the majority of revision was restricted to online, web-based practice questions. The availability of written resources focussing on the principles of the MRCPsych syllabus was limited and poorly presented. The texts were often wordy, and the graphics were overly complicated. It was difficult to pick out key learning points and to identify what was relevant to passing the exams.

Whilst the online questions banks are an appropriate strategy for passing the written papers, there are times when we wanted to study but didn't have access to the internet or didn't want to be staring at a screen. It is for those reasons we have written this book, with Bhaskar Punukollu's support. It is intended to be concise where appropriate and to present information using graphics where possible. It is pocket sized so it can be pulled out at a moment's notice. We hope you find it a useful addition to your learning.

Good luck!

DOI: 10.1201/9781003322573-1

Part I

Behavioural Sciences and Sociocultural Psychiatry

1 Fundamentals of Psychology

Elizabeth Templeton

a) Conditioning

Conditioning is the process of increasing the likelihood of a behavioural response in an individual by reinforcement using a stimulus or a reward.

Classical Conditioning

The work of Ivan **Pavlov**:[1]

Classical condition is concerned with *responses to a stimulus* whereas operant conditioning is concerned with *responses to behaviour*.

Classical conditioning is produced by *pairing* a conditioned stimulus such as a bell with a natural (unconditioned) stimulus (UCS) such as food. The natural stimulus will produce a natural response such as salivation; however, if the conditioned stimulus (CS) (bell) and the unconditioned stimulus (food) are repeatedly paired and presented together, then eventually the bell alone will evoke the desired response, now the conditioned response of salivation.

Pavlov demonstrated this using dogs.

Food = salivation
Bell + food = salivation
Bell alone = salivation

The development of a conditioned response (CR) from a conditioned stimulus is called *acquisition* and can be a relatively quick process. Different types of conditioning are explained in Table 1.1.

Thorndike's Law of Effect[2]

Edward Thorndike's law of effect states that the tendency of an action to occur depends on the effect it has on the environment.

Operant Conditioning[3]

Operant conditioning is the work of B. F. **Skinner**. This theory of learning suggests people *learn by interacting* (operating) with their environment.

DOI: 10.1201/9781003322573-3

Table 1.1 Different types of conditioning and important terms

Term	Description
Simultaneous conditioning	CS (bell) and UCS (food) are presented together.
Backward conditioning	UCS presented first, followed by the CS.
Forward (delayed) conditioning	CS presented first, followed by the UCS.
Trace conditioning	CS is presented but then stopped prior to the presentation of the UCS—conditioning reliant on *memory trace.*
Temporal condition	Here the UCS is paired to *time*. So, if food is presented to the dog every hour, the dog will eventually start to salivate (CR) just prior to the presentation of food.
Higher order conditioning	This refers to the use of a *CS being used as the UCS* and being paired with a new CS—for example, once the bell evokes the CR saliva, it becomes the UCS, and the bell could then be paired with new CS such as a whistle.
Stimulus generalisation	This is the extension of the CR—for example, if the CS is a white rat and the CR is fear, this could generalise into a fear of all small white animals or even objects.
Extinction	If the CS is repeatedly presented without the UCS, then the *CR will disappear.*
Spontaneous recovery	If the UCS is then presented with the CS, the *CR can return* to some degree.
Counter conditioning	*Replacing a previous CR with a new CR*—for example, if a dog has learned to bark at the postman every day, you might try and teach it a new behaviour, such as sitting quietly.
Incubation	*Increased strength of the CR* when repeatedly exposed to the CS.
Stimulus preparedness	Phobias are more likely to develop to a stimulus we are hard wired to fear, such as snakes.

Table 1.2 The principles of reinforcement and punishment

Term	Description
Positive reinforcer	Desirable response *given* (food given after pressing a bell).
Negative reinforcer	Undesirable experience *taken away* (cessation of electric shock after pressing bell).
Positive punishment	Undesirable response *given* (naughty child has to sit on the naughty step).
Negative punishment	Desirable response *taken away* (paying a fine).
Primary reinforcer	Relates to biological needs such as food/water and sex.
Secondary reinforcer	A.k.a. conditioned reinforcers, in other words, people have to learn to like them, such as social approval or money.

Operant conditioning relies on the principle of *reinforcement and punishment*. Reinforcement aims to increase the frequency of a behaviour, whereas punishment is used to decrease the frequency of a behaviour. Both reinforcement and punishment can be positive or negative (Table 1.2).

Operant conditioning involves an organism learning an appropriate behaviour because it is followed by a desirable consequence. This is the basis of reinforcement and how we learn by trial and error. The phenomena itself is called *the law of effect* and is often demonstrated by Thorndike's experiments. A condition that leads to a decrease of behaviour following learning is known as punishment.

Reinforcement schedules:

*   **Fixed interval**—a reward after a fixed amount of time regardless of number of responses.
*   **Variable interval**—a reward after a varying unpredictable amount of time.
*   **Fixed ratio**—a reward occurs after a behaviour is repeated x number of times, for example, the rat is given a treat after it presses the lever five times.
*   **Variable ratio**—a reward occurs after a random number of responses.
*   **Random**—no pattern.

Fixed schedules favour learning:

Variable schedules take longer to learn but are harder to extinct. Gambling mimics variable ratio reinforcement, hence, why gambling addiction is so hard to treat. Types of conditioning are defined in Table 1.3.

Table 1.3 Types of conditioning

Type of conditioning	Definition
Aversive conditioning	Where a *negative stimulus* is paired with an *unwanted behaviour*: for example, the use of disulfiram in alcohol abuse.
Premack's principle/ Grandma's rule	An existing *high frequency* behaviour is used to *enhance* a *low frequency* but desirable behaviour: for example, eat all of your vegetables, and you can have your dessert.
Covert reinforcement	An *imaginary desirable response* is used to as the positive reinforcement: for example, imagining passing all of your exams with 100% to help with your revision.
Covert sensitisation	An *imaginary undesirable response* is used to reduce a certain behaviour: for example, an alcoholic might imagine getting fired to try to reduce his drinking pattern.
Avoidance learning	Avoiding a certain experience to produce a desirable effect: for example, agoraphobic patients avoid open spaces to reduce their anxiety. This can often be hard to reverse.
Flooding	*Abrupt exposure* to a feared stimulus until the fear response has subsided: for example, asking a person with a spider phobia to hold a tarantula until they no longer feel scared. This can be counterproductive if the person leaves before the fear response has subsided and becomes more fearful of the stimulus.

b) Shaping and Chaining

Shaping

Otherwise known as *successive approximations* where approximation of the desired behaviour is reinforced. This might be used when training animals to perform certain tricks for TV or perhaps in the circus.

> Tiger runs towards a hoop—gets a treat.
> Then, tiger runs towards hoop then through it—gets a treat.
> Then, tiger runs towards hoop and runs and jumps through—gets a treat.
> Finally, tiger runs through hoop set on fire—behaviour achieved.

Chaining

The new desired behaviour might be a *series of successive behaviours*. Each behaviour is the cue for the next, and the last produces a reinforcement.

For example, a child learning the alphabet or tying shoelaces.

Reinforcement occurs once the child has mastered the whole task.

Learned Helplessness

The theory states that when an organism is confronted with *an aversive stimulus* from which it is *impossible to escape*, it will *stop trying*. This was demonstrated experimentally using dogs placed in a room and given an electric shock through the floor. Initially the dog would try and get out of the room, but eventually the dog stops trying to escape.

This has been suggested as model for depression or domestic violence when the individual seems unable to help themselves.

c) Social Learning Theory[4]

Social learning theory is based on work by Albert **Bandura**, who provided an alternative theory to learning via reinforcement. He proposed that individuals could *learn by observation alone.*

Social learning theory emphasises the role of cognition and states that people learn by a variety of mechanisms and their learning is affected by factors such as *goal seeking, appraisal* and *striving for meaning.*

Reciprocal Causation

Bandura proposed that the behaviour, the environment and the individual all influence each other.

Bandura's Bobo Doll Experiment

Children were shown a model that acted aggressively towards a doll. They were later observed to repeat the aggression towards the doll without any reinforcement.

Children are particularly *susceptible to observational learning* from caregivers.

Insight Learning

Learning is proposed to be a *purely cognitive* process and not based on a stimulus-response mechanism.

Cognitive Learning

Reinforcement might be needed for a performance of a learned response but not necessarily for the learning to occur (latent learning).

d) Perceptual Organisation

Figure vs. Ground Differentiation[5]

Generally, when we look at something, for example, seeing a friend in the park, the person will be emphasised (figure) over the trees, grass and bench (ground).

Gestalt Principle of Perceptual Organisation[6]

- **Similarity**—items that look similar will be group together based on colour or shape.
- **Proximity**—two items close together will be perceived as one.
- **Closure**—people tend to fill in missing contours to perceive a whole shape.
- **Common fate**—items that move together are perceived as one object.
- **Continuity**—items that form a continuous shape are perceives as belonging together.
- **Pragnanz**—this is the basis of Gestalt's theory, stating that every stimulus pattern is seen in the most structurally simplistic way.

Perception of Depth Distance and Motion[7]

This is made possible by *stimulus cues*, which can be either pictorial or non-pictorial.

Pictorial cues include size, brightness, texture, liner perspective, superimposition, aerial perspective and motion parallax.

Non-pictorial cues include things such as retinal image disparity, stereopsis, accommodation and convergence.

Depth and distance perception are abnormal in:

- Temporal lobe epilepsy
- Derealisation
- Acute brain injury
- Schizophrenia

Perceptual constancy is the ability to perceive objects as being the same despite variation in position/angle; a door is a door regardless of the angle it is at.

Phi phenomenon,[8] noted by Max **Wertheimer**, states that images shown in a rapid sequence create the impression of motion. Motion pictures are based on this principle.

Autokinesis[9] refers to the phenomenon that if a light source is shown in a dark room for a prolonged period of time, the light will appear as if it is moving. This visual illusion can affect pilots and can also be an explanation for UFO sightings.

e) Theories of Perception[10,11]

Top-Down Theory

Retinal images can not alone be responsible for the perceptions we experience. Perception is a *mix of higher cortical processing* what we already know and *understanding* or making sense of the retinal images.

Bottom-Up Theory

Gestalt law is an example of bottom-up theory; perception is driven by the *optic array*. Piecing together the basic elements of an image triggers more complex higher cortical systems.

f) Memory[12,13,14]

Memory is the ability to *store, retain and retrieve information.*

Three different processes are thought to occur:

Encoding/registration is the initial formation of memory. It can be visual, acoustic or semantic and can be improved by organising data, for example, using mnemonics.

Storage is either short-term:

- **Short-term memory (STM)**, according to George **Miller** (1956), is usually stated as 7 ± 2 (the average person can remember seven numbers consecutively). This can be assisted by chunking the information together.

- STM will be lost in about *18 seconds* if rehearsal or repetition don't take place soon after; however, if utilised, STM can be extended for an indefinite period of time.
- Information coded *visually feeds sooner than auditory* coding.

Or long-term:

- **Long-term memory (LTM)** can last from *minutes to a lifetime*. The coding is largely semantic (with meaning added) but can be visual or acoustic.
- *Rehearsal* can transfer memories from STM to LTM. Rehearsal may be maintenance and repetitive or elaborate and semantic.
- Long-term memory requires *consolidation* and must be left undisturbed for a few minutes. Major disruption such as a head injury can lead to retrograde amnesia.

g) Retrieval

Retrieval in STM is normally effortless and error free. It can be affected by *primacy*, *latency* and *serial position* (items at the beginning and end are remembered better than items in the middle).

Recall appears to be organised according to applied strategies such as *semantic clustering*.

When a memory can be affected by a person's *internal* state, it is called *state dependent*.

When memory can be affected by an individual's *environment*, it can be considered *context dependent*.

Other classifications:

Memory can be classified according to whether it can be consciously and intentionally retrieved: either *declarative* (explicit) or *non-declarative* (implicit).

Declarative memories can be further divided into:

- **Semantic fact based**—factual knowledge, for example, grass is green.
- **Episodic event based**—autobiographical, self-focussed.

Non-Declarative (Implicit Memory)

- **Procedural**—such as driving a car.
- **Priming**—the episode of learning cannot be recalled, but performance demonstrates that the information is learned.

Summary

The major systems of memory are summarised in Table 1.4.

Table 1.4 Major systems of memory

Major system	Other terms	Retrieval
1. Procedural	Non-declarative	Implicit
2. Perceptual representation	Quasi-memory	Implicit
3. Short-term	Primary, working	Explicit
4. Semantic	Knowledge	Implicit
5. Episodic	Autobiographical	Explicit

Working Memory[15]

Alan **Baddeley** and Graham **Hitch** (1974) were unimpressed with the theory of short-term memory, believing it to be too simplistic. They produced a new concept—*working memory*.

Working memory is short-term memory, but rather than all the information going into a single store with relatively little processing, a different system was proposed for different types of information. Baddeley and Hitch introduced the idea that the working memory had a central executive function, controlling and coordinating an operation in two subsystems. Think of it as the boss!

- **The phonological loop**—deals with spoken and written word; it uses auditory rehearsal loops.
- **Visuospatial sketch pad**—stores and processes information in a visual or spatial form.
- **The episodic buffer**—acts as a 'backup' store, which communicates with both long-term memory and the components of working memory.

Forgetting

- Rapid loss of acquired information.
- Forgetting is *maximum in the first few hours* after learning; it is never complete, with some information always retained.
- It can be influenced by activity between learning and recall.
- New information can displace older information, or a piece of information can make storing or recalling other information more difficult.
- *Retroactive interference*: new information can interfere with the recall of old information
- *Pro-active interference*: past learning is likely to impair rather than aid subsequent learning.

Decay theory states that forgetting is *time dependent*, so forgetting is due to disuse of the memory over time; there is no evidence of neurological decay, and what happened before and after learning appears to be more important than just the passage of time.

h) Ribot's Law[16]

Théodule-Armand **Ribot** suggested that recent memories might be more vulnerable to brain injury than remote memories.

Ribot observed that people who suffer traumatic events often lose the memory leading up to the event.

The saying goes '*you lose first what you learned last*'.

The same is seen in patients with Alzheimer's disease. This might be related to the dependence of retrieval on the hippocampal systems.

i) Memory Disorders[17]

* **Amnesia**—pure memory deficit.
* **Retrograde amnesia**—loss of memory for past events *prior to the lesion* occurring.
* **Anterograde amnesia**—inability to make new memories *from the time of the lesion*.
* **Transient global amnesia** (TGA)—the sudden loss of *predominantly anterograde and variable retrograde* memory. Memory loss is *transient* and can't be attributed to a neurological condition.
* *Brief episodes* of memory loss suggest **transient epileptic amnesia** (TEA).

Note that dissociative memory loss is *not an organic syndrome* but occurs as part of a dissociative fugue. It is normally retrograde and episodic, relating to an event or period of time. The forgotten events are usually *traumatic*.

j) Memory Neuroscience[18,19]

Short-term memory depends on the *electrical actions* of neurons.

Long-term memory results from *changes to the neural circuit*, such as changes in synapses or branching of dendrites and increased neuroglial cells.

k) Brain Structures Involved in Memory[20,21]

The **amygdala** is thought to *regulate the emotional* importance of an experience and hippocampal activity.

It is involved in emotional memory and emotional face processing.

Damage can lead to loss of maternal instincts in monkeys and loss of fear conditioning.

The **hippocampus** is linked with regions of the *temporal lobe* and *prefrontal cortex*, and is responsible for the coding and retrieval of information.

The *left* hippocampus encodes *verbal declarative* memory and the *right*, *non-verbal* memories.

Damage to the hippocampus can result in anterograde amnesia; however, unilateral lesions are normally well compensated for, and amnesia does not occur.

Damage to the *hypothalamus*, *mammillary bodies* and terminal portions of the *hippocampus* can give risk to *Korsakoff-like* memory loss.

Notes

1. Pavlov, I. P. (1928). *Lectures on Conditioned Reflexes* (W. H. Gantt, Trans.). London: Allen and Unwin.
2. Thorndike, E. L. (1898). Animal Intelligence: An Experimental Study of the Associative Processes in Animals. *Psychological Monographs: General and Applied,* 2 (4): i–109.
3. Ferster, C. B., and B. F. Skinner. (1957). *Schedules of Reinforcement.* New York: Appleton-Century-Crofts.
4. Bandura, A. (1977). *Social Learning Theory.* Englewood Cliffs, NJ: Prentice Hall.
5. Rubin, E. (2001). Figure and Ground. In S. Yantis (Ed.), *Visual Perception.* Philadelphia, PA: Psychology Press, pp. 225–229.
6. Humphrey, G. (1924). The Psychology of the Gestalt. *Journal of Educational Psychology,* 15 (7): 401–412. doi:10.1037/h0070207.
7. Howard, I. (2012). *Perceiving in Depth.* New York: Oxford University Press.
8. Wertheimer, M. (1912, April). *Experimentelle Studien über das Sehen von Bewegung.* Leipzig: Johann Ambrosius Barth Publishing House.
9. Gregory, R. L. (1977). *Eye and Brain: The Psychology of Seeing.* 3rd ed. London: Weidenfeld & Nicolson, p. 105.
10. Goldstein, E. B. (13 February 2009). *Sensation and Perception.* Belmont, CA: Cengage Learning.
11. Gregory, R. L., and O. L. Zangwill. (1987). *The Oxford Companion to the Mind.* Oxford: Oxford University Press.
12. Matlin, M. W. (2005). *Cognition.* Crawfordsville: John Wiley & Sons, Inc.
13. Miller, G. A. (1956). The Magical Number Seven, Plus or Minus Two: Some Limits on Our Capacity for Processing Information. *Psychological Review,* 63 (2): 81–97.
14. Sternberg, R. J. (1999). *Cognitive Psychology.* 2nd ed. Fort Worth, TX: Harcourt Brace College Publishers.
15. Baddeley, A. D., and G. Hitch. (1974). Working Memory. In G. H. Bower (Ed.), *The Psychology of Learning and Motivation: Advances in Research and Theory.* New York: Academic Press, Vol. 8, pp. 47–89.
16. Wixted, J. T. (2004, October). On Common Ground: Jost's (1897) Law of Forgetting and Ribot's (1881) Law of Retrograde Amnesia. *Psychological Review,* 111 (4): 864–879.
17. Kopelman, M. D. (2002). Disorders of Memory. *Brain,* 125 (10): 2152–2190.
18. Jacobsen, C. F. (1938). Studies of Cerebral Function in Primates. *Comp Psychological Monographs,* 13: 1–68.
19. Ashby, F. G., S. W. Ell, V. V. Valentin, and M. B. Casale. (2005, November). FROST: A Distributed Neurocomputational Model of Working Memory Maintenance. *Journal of Cognitive Neuroscience,* 17 (11): 1728–1743.
20. Barbey, A. K., M. Koenigs, and J. Grafman. (2013). Dorsolateral Prefrontal Contributions to Human Working Memory. *Cortex,* 49 (5): 1195–1205.
21. Owen, A. M. (1997, July). The Functional Organization of Working Memory Processes Within Human Lateral Frontal Cortex: The Contribution of Functional Neuroimaging. *The European Journal of Neuroscience,* 9 (7): 1329–1339.

2 Basic and Social Psychology

Elizabeth Templeton

a) Personality
b) Emotion
c) Motivation
d) Attitudes
e) Intelligence
f) Cognitive Dissonance (Leon Festinger)
g) Self-Psychology
h) Attribution
i) Theory of Mind
j) Controversial Studies
k) Groups and Conforming
l) Consent in Minors

a) Personality

Consider the Differing Concepts of Personality

The idiographic view assumes that each person has a unique personality, parts of which can only be possessed by that individual and cannot be directly compared to another. The following quotes are examples of an idiographic view:

> Personality is the dynamic organization within the individual of those psychophysical systems that determine his characteristics behaviour and thoughts.[1]
> The characteristics or blend of characteristics that make a person unique.[2]

The nomothetic view assumes that personality traits have the same psychological meaning in everyone, although some people might differ along the continuum of one trait; therefore, people can be compared.

DOI: 10.1201/9781003322573-4

Freud's Theory

Sigmund **Freud**'s psychodynamic model assumes there is an interaction between nature and nurture in personality development.

The Structural Model

> **Id**—the primitive and instinctive component of personality; contains the libido instinct (*Eros*) and the death instinct (Thanatos). The Id operates on the pleasure principle.
>
> **Ego**—mediates between the will of the Id and the outside world to aid in our decision making. It operates according to the reality principle.
>
> **Superego (psyche)**—represents the morals of society, which are learned from our parents. It can punish the Id with feelings of guilt and can be thought of as our conscience.[3]

Alternative Theories

Trait Theory[4]

- Traits are the fundamental units of personality.
- People differ with regard to how much of a trait they possess, which can result in an endless number of different personalities.
- Traits should remain consistent across situations and over time, explaining why people behave in a predictable way in different settings.
- These theories measure personality based on psychometric tests and are sometimes referred to as psychometric theories because of this.

Allport's Theory[5]

Gordon **Allport** (1961) believed that people have core central traits which are usually apparent to others and affect that person's behaviour, for example, being excitable or reliable.

In general, people have approximately five to ten central traits.

Allport believed that people also have secondary traits; these are more specific, that only a close friend might notice and might only influence a few behaviours, for example, does not like big crowds.

Cattell's 16 Personality Factor Approach[6]

Raymond **Cattell** (1957) collected data from a range of different sources:

> **L data**—life record, school performance, work absences, etc.
> **Q data**—questionnaires designed to rate an individual's personality.
> **T data**—data from objective tests.

Cattell used factor analysis to determine the degree to which these traits correlated with each other.

He identified 16 traits common to all people.

He divided these traits into surface traits that are very obvious to all people, and source traits, which are more subtle. Source traits influence several aspects of a person's behaviour and were regarded as more important in determining their personality.

Cattell produced a personality test, the 16 PF personality factors test, which has 160 questions in total, with ten questions relating to each factor.

Eysenck's Approach[7]

Hans **Eysenck** (1975) interviewed soldiers and found that behaviour could be represented by two dimensions: 'introversion/extroversion' and 'neuroticism/ stability'.

According to Eysenck, these two dimensions could combine to form a variety of personality characteristics:

* Extraverts
* Introverts
* Neurotic unstables
* Stables

Later he added a 'psychoticism' dimension—lacking empathy, cruelty, loner, rejects social norms.

Eysenck believed that a person's personality was related to their autonomic nervous system and was determined by the balance of excitation and inhibition.

The 'Big Five' Personality Traits[8]

Described by Robert R. **McCrae** and Paul **Costa Jr.** (1992) as:

* Openness
* Conscientiousness
* Extraversion
* Agreeableness
* Neuroticism

Measuring Personality Traits

There are two main types of personality tests: projective and objective tests.

Examples of projective tests include:

* Rorschach Inkblot
* Thematic Apperception test

- Draw-A-Person test
- Sentence completion tests

Projective tests are designed to assess unconscious material. In principle, by presenting individuals with ambiguous shapes or pictures, they will reveal hidden emotions and conflicts by projecting them into the tests.

Objective tests have very structured and clear questions and aims.

Examples of objective tests include:

- Minnesota Multiphasic Personality Inventory
- Sixteen Personality Factor Questionnaire (16PF)
- NEO Personality Inventory
- Eysenck Personality Test (EPQ)

b) Emotion

There are six primary human emotions identified by Paul **Ekman** (1969);[9] surprise, fear, sadness, anger, happiness and disgust.

Four main theories of emotion come up in membership exams:

- James-Lange theory
- Cannon-Bard theory
- Singer-Schachter theory
- Lazarus theory

The key to understanding the difference between these is being clear where the stimulus for the emotion arises.

James-Lange Theory[10]

Emotion is the result of bodily changes. For example, if you see a wild lion, your heart starts to race, your palms become sweaty and these peripheral responses send feedback to the cortex, and you interpret this as fear.

The sequence of events proposed was as follows:

Event—arousal—interpretation—emotion
The stimulus for emotion arises from physical sensations.

Cannon-Bard Theory (a.k.a. Thalami Theory)[11]

This theory proposed that information about an emotional situation is sent to the thalamus, which simultaneously sends information to the cortex and to the autonomic nervous system.

The brain creates the emotion.

Singer-Schachter Theory (a.k.a. Two-Factor Theory)[12]

This theory suggests that emotions result from cognitive interpretations of the physiological changes. For example, if one's heart is racing whilst on a first date, one is labelled as excited; but if one's heart is racing whilst at the top of a roller-coaster, one is labelled as afraid.

The stimulus for emotion arises via a combination of physical sensations and the mind's evaluation of them.

Lazarus Theory[13]

This theory suggests that a thought is first required before an emotion occurs. For example, you see a large snake; you think it is going to bite you and you feel scared.

The stimulus for emotion arises from the mind.

c) Motivation

Maslow's Hierarchy of Needs[14]

Abraham **Maslow** (1943) proposed a hierarchy of human needs as a way of explaining motivation (Figure 2.1).

At the bottom of the pyramid are human biological needs; a person cannot progress further up the pyramid until basic needs are met. Once the basic needs are met, these will no longer be prioritised and the individual will focus

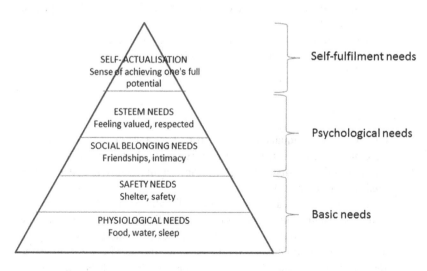

Figure 2.1 Maslow's hierarchy of needs

on meeting the higher-level needs. If at any point one of the lower-level sets of needs is no longer being met, this will temporarily be prioritised once again.

d) Attitudes

Martin **Fishbein** and Icek **Ajzen** (1975) defined attitudes as:

Learned predispositions to respond in a consistently favourable or unfavourable way towards a given object person or event.[15]

(p. 6)

Attitudes can be thought of as a combination of beliefs and values.

Beliefs are objective and link an object to an attribute based on knowledge of the world; for example, animals are integral to the environment.

Values are subjective and relate to your personal feelings regarding the object; for example, the value 'harming animals is not acceptable' can turn into an attitude: 'I will not eat meat'.

Attitudes have three key features:

* **Cognitive**—vegetables and fruits are good for me and give me energy.
* **Affective**—health is very important to me.
* **Behavioural**—I always eat a healthy diet.

Daniel **Katz** (1960) described the functions of attitudes:[16]

1. **Social adjustment**—help us to fit in with or belong to a group.
2. **Ego defensive**—act as a defence for personal deficiencies. These types of attitudes are often very hard to change.
3. **Knowledge function**—help us make sense of the world.
4. **Value expressive**—allow us to express ourselves, for example, vegetarianism.

Attitude Scales[17]

Likert scale—Individuals are asked to rate their level of agreement to a statement by circling usually one of five answers ranging from strongly agree to strongly disagree. This is one of the simplest and preferred methods of rating attitudes.

Thurstone scale—Created by a panel of judges. Subjects are given a number of statements pertaining to a specific topic and they must rate each statement. Twenty statements, both negative and positive, are then assigned to that topic based on the previous rating. These 20 statements form an attitude scale. This method of measuring attitude is generally not used, as it is tedious and complicated.

Osgood's Semantic Differential

This is a 7-point scale, each point on the scale represented by opposing labels (strong-weak, good-bad).

For example, one might wish to compare a person of interest such as a politician. This scale allows for opposing attitudes to be measured on the same scale by using bipolar labels.

Each individual could have any score from 1 (honest) to 7 (dishonest), with a score of 3–4 being neutral.

Guttman scale—items are ranked in a cumulative fashion; agreeing to a higher ranked item indicates that you agree to the lower ranked items also.

For example: 'I am willing to be near meat', 'I am willing to smell meat', 'I am willing to cook meat', 'I am willing to eat meat'.

Another use of this type of scale might be to record abilities of achievements; for example, if a student can multiply two-digit numbers 10×20, then one could assume that the same student could multiply one-digit numbers 5×5.

e) Intelligence

Louis Leon **Thurstone** argued that intelligence could not be measured by a single factor. He further argued that intelligence arises from seven independent factors he called primary abilities:[18]

- Word fluency
- Verbal comprehension
- Spatial visualisation
- Number facility
- Associative memory
- Reasoning
- Perceptual speed

The National Adult Reading Test (NART)

This is used to test the pre-morbid intelligence levels of English speakers. It is commonly used in patients with dementia.

f) Cognitive Dissonance (Leon Festinger[19])

In general, people aim to hold beliefs that are congruent with their actions; however, cognitive dissonance (conflict) allows a person to hold two differing beliefs in their consciousness simultaneously.

A good example is people who smoke tobacco (behaviour) are often aware that cigarettes are harmful but continue to smoke (dissonance/conflict).

The theory suggests that we all have an inner drive towards cognitive consistency so that beliefs and behaviours exist in harmony. In order to adapt, we might create new cognitions which help assimilate the two that are in dissonance; 'it will never happen to me'.

Dissonance can be reduced in a number of ways:

- One or more attitudes, behaviours or beliefs can be changed.
- New information can be acquired.
- The importance of the cognitions can be reduced.

g) Self-Psychology

Self-psychology encompasses various different concepts:

- **Self-esteem**—the attitude one holds towards themselves that reflects their worthiness.
- **Self-consciousness**—the awareness of the self in comparison to others. Something thought only to be associated with the human race.
- **Self-image**—is often a combination of physical attributes, personality traits and social roles.

Gordon **Gallup Jr.**'s (1970)[20] 'touching the dot' experiment aimed to demonstrate when self-recognition had been developed.

A red dot is placed on a child's forehead and then the child is placed in front of a mirror and observed to see if they start searching their face to find the dot.

From 5–25% of infants attempt to touch the dot by searching their own face by 18 months, and 75% of children touch the dot by 20 months. Thus, self-recognition develops between the ages of 18–20 months.

Mirror recognition demonstrated by primates is different. Primates are able to identify that what they see in the mirror is the same as them, but are unable to recognise the image as them.

h) Attribution

Attribution is the process in which we make judgements about the cause of behaviours.

As humans, it is important for individuals to attempt an understanding of the actions of others, so we piece information together to reach a reasonable conclusion. However, in doing this, we often introduce bias (Table 2.1), which leads us to inaccurate inferences regarding human behaviour.

Other factors known to affect behaviour include:

Hawthorne effect, a.k.a. the observer effect—there is short-term improvement in behaviour/efficiency when being watched.

Table 2.1 Types of bias

Fundamental attribution error
This refers to overestimating character traits and minimising external factors as an explanation for behaviour. This occurs commonly in substances misuse: 'that person takes drug because they are bad/immoral', rather than considering the circumstances.

Self-serving bias (SSB)
Refers to the tendency to attribute positive behaviours to internal factors: 'I did well on that test because I am clever' and negative behaviours to external causes: 'I failed my tests because the room was too hot'.
Depressed people do not tend to demonstrate SSB and are overly self-critical.

Actor observer effect
When comparing our behaviour to others, we have a tendency to attribute external factors to our own behaviours: 'I drink because I am having a difficult time' and other people's behaviour to internal factors: 'he drinks because he is a weak person'.

Just world hypothesis
This refers to the belief that we live in a just world, and therefore if something bad happened to you, then you must be a bad person or deserving. This can lead to victim blaming.

False consensus effect
This is a tendency to view the behaviour of one of a few individuals as representative of the entire group. This can lead to racial and cultural stereotypes.

- **Primacy effect**—first impressions are often heavily weighted when meeting a stranger. A positive first impression is more likely to change than a negative first impression.
- **Halo effect**—assuming that a person is wholly good based on a few superficial attributes such as looks. This can be seen in reverse, particularly by the police who might view a person as wholly bad or guilty because they share the attributes of other criminals.
- **Pygmalion effect**—self-fulfilling prophecy: if a teacher criticises a student and labels them as bad, they are more likely to identify with this label and perform poorly academically.

i) Theory of Mind

Theory of mind is the understanding that others have beliefs/thought/feelings distinct from our own.

It develops around 3–4 years of age.

In some disorders such as autism, there might be a deficit in theory if mind development. In others, such as acute psychosis, there might be a transient deficit in theory of mind.[21]

Sally Anne Test

Devised by Simon **Baron-Cohen**[22] to test the **theory of the mind**.

The study included a group of 60 children with a diagnosis of autism, Down syndrome or unimpaired.

The children were introduced to two characters, Sally and Anne, and shown a short skit, as in Figure 2.2. Sally takes a marble and places it into her basket and then leaves. Anne enters and removes Sally's marble and puts it into her own box. The children are then asked the belief question, 'Where will Sally look for the marble?'

The researchers found that the autistic children answered 'in the box': they failed to understand that Sally would have a different understanding to themselves of where the marble might be.

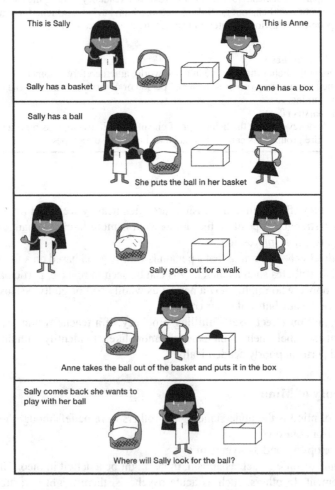

Figure 2.2 Sally Anne Test

Linguistics

The four core components of language are:

- **Semantics**—analyses the connection between language and meanings. Is meaning inherent in language, or does the meaning depend on how the individual is speaking?
- **Pragmatics**—studies the way in which context contributes to meaning.
- **Syntax**—the study of sentence structure.
- **Phonology**—studies the organisation of sounds in language.

Methods of Persuasive Communication

- **Arousal of guilt.**
- **Reciprocity**—offering or completing a favour prior to asking.
- **Scarcity**—'running out fast, get yours quick'.
- **Ingratiation**—befriending.
- **Social validation**—everybody else has one.
- **'Foot in the door' technique**—make a smaller request prior to asking larger request.
- **'Door in the face' technique**—ask for a large request; when that is turned down, they maybe more likely to consent to a smaller request.

j) Controversial Studies

Stanford Prison Experiment[23]
This study looked at how people adapt to given roles. A mock prison was set up and 24 students were recruited; they were split into two groups: prisoner or guard.
They were given no guidance on how to behave, except the guards were told not to use any physical violence and they were told they could terminate the experiment if they chose.
Within a short space of time, the participants began to identify with their roles and the guards devised cruel and harsh punishments for the prisoners. After six days, some of the prisoners showed signs of emotional distress and the study had to be terminated.

The Tuskegee Syphilis Experiment[24]
This infamous study aimed to follow the natural progression of syphilis. The study recruited mainly impoverished African-American men. The participants were never told their diagnosis and were never given penicillin, even after it had become widely available as a treatment for syphilis.
Furthermore, participants were actively prevented from seeking treatment that had become available to other residents. Numerous participants died and passed on the diseases to their wives; 19 children were born with congenital syphilis.
The study was shut down after whistle-blowers came forward. It led to major changes in US law and regulations related to ethical research.

(Continued)

(Continued)

The Tearooms Study[25]
The study was conducted by Laud **Humphreys**, an American sociologist with an
  interest in researching sexual encounters between homosexual men.
Humphreys would hang around 'tea-rooms'—public toilets where sexual encounters
  would take place—and interview the men or observe their sexual encounters. This
  was done under the guise of voyeurism, and Humphreys never told these men he
  was conducting research.
This study raised questions around informed consent.

Milgram's Study[26]
This study was started shortly after the Second World War, when many Nazi soldiers
  stood trial for war crimes. The public were shocked and appalled by the German
  soldiers' treatment of the Jewish people in Germany. However, many of the soldiers
  defended their actions by stating they were just following orders.
Stanley **Milgram** set out to see if participants from a diverse range of backgrounds
  would follow orders and perform acts that may cause injury and distress to others.
  They found unexpectedly that a very high proportion of people would do so.
The participants were given the role of a teacher and told there was another volunteer
  who played the role of a learner; however, this was not a volunteer but somebody
  working for the trial.
Every time the learner gave an incorrect answer, the teacher was told to administer a
  shock to the learner. They could not see the learner, but they could hear them, so the
  subjects believed the learner was actually receiving a shock. In reality, this was not
  the case. The shocks became progressively stronger.
The learner would occasionally scream in pain following a shock. If
  a subject showed a desire to stop the experiment, they were given a series of
  non-threatening verbal prompts. In total, 65% of the volunteers administered the
  maximum shock of 450 volts, much higher than anybody had predicted at the start
  of the study.

The Willowbrook Study[27]
This study was designed to assess the effects of gamma globulin on hepatitis.
  The study took place at the Willowbrook institute for children with learning
  disabilities.
The researchers were accused of purposefully injecting healthy children with hepatitis
  and then treating them with gamma globulin to monitor the potential as a new
  treatment.

---

k) Groups and Conforming

Solomon Asch Conformity Experiment[28]

Solomon **Asch** wanted to explore the effect that a person's willingness to want
to conform in group scenario would have on their behaviour.

Asch told his subjects that they were anticipating a visual perception task
(Figure 2.3). He put the subjects into groups of eight to ten people. In each
group there was only one real subject, with the others being researchers in the
study posing as other subjects.

Asch would then show the group this diagram and ask them to which line
exhibit 1 was closest in length, from A, B and C. The group was asked to

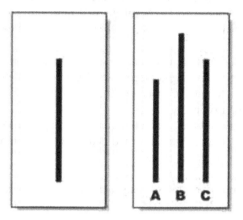

Figure 2.3 Solomon Asch Conformity Experiment

state their answer aloud, with the subject answering last. It was repeated at least 18 times. The researcher subjects would give a deliberately wrong answer. Asch found that the majority of the true subjects would also give a wrong answer.

Asch concluded that people conformed for two main reasons:

- They think the group is better informed than they are.
- They want to be liked by the group.

Group Psychology

Wilfred Bion

Wilfred **Bion** was a psychoanalyst who is well known for his observations on 'group dynamics'.

Bion also coined the term 'containing', which refers to the ability of a person or service to absorb another person's projection.

Bion argued that a group is normally split into the working group and the basic assumption group.

The working group focusses on accomplishing the primary task of the group.

The basic assumption group describes the underlying assumptions of the group that influence the way it behaves.[29]

Bion described three basic assumptions:

- **Dependency**—the group looks for a leader to provide security and protect them from anxiety. The leader is idealised by the group. Some individuals are more susceptible to this role than others; however, the group can start to resent the leader and find a replacement. In situ, this might be demonstrated by a group who meets for the first time and sits in silence until somebody nominates themselves to break the ice and becomes a leader figure.

- **Fight-flight**—the group unites against a common enemy. This might be shown by aggression (fight), seen in rivalry between football clubs. Or if the enemy is internal, the group might act out (flight) by chatting amongst themselves or arriving late.
- **Pairing**—works on the assumption that the group will be stronger if two of its members are paired. The two people will then more successfully drive the group to complete its work.

Working in groups can bring many benefits, but potential problems can occur:

- Groupthink
- Groupshift
- Deindividuation

Groupthink

Groupthink[30] is a term coined by Irving **Janis** in 1972.

It occurs when a group of people make poor or irrational decisions because of the pressure to conform or succeed. The group will try and reach a consensus agreement without asking critical questions.

Groupthink is most likely to happen when the group is insulated from outside opinions, its members share similar backgrounds and there is a culture of loyalty and inflated confidence within the group.

Symptoms of groupthink include:

- Stereotypes of 'out-groups'.
- Belief in the inherent morality of the group.
- Illusion of invulnerability.
- Collective rationalisation.
- Self-censorship.
- Direct pressure on dissenters: it is discouraged to question the groups views.
- Self-appointed mind guards: members who take it upon themselves to protect the group and the leader from problematic information.
- Illusion of unanimity: it is assumed that everybody agrees with the decision being made.

Poor decisions made by cohesive groups of politicians might be considered examples of groupthink. Janis names several examples, such as the failure to anticipate the Pearl Harbour attack and the invasion occurring during the Iraq war.

In order to prevent groupthink, the following principles should be applied to group decision making:

- Outside experts should be allowed to attend meetings.
- Leaders should encourage each member to challenge ideas and present objections.
- The leader should avoid expressing opinions about their preferred outcome.
- Members should talk about and solicit ideas with people outside the group.
- The group should assign a 'devil's advocate' at all meetings to challenge any and all ideas.[31]

Groupshift

Groupshift is the phenomenon in which the initial positions of individual members of a group are exaggerated towards a more extreme position. For example, when people are in groups, they assess risk differently than they do when they are alone. In the group, they are likely to make riskier decisions, as the shared risk makes the individual risk seem to be less.

One Example of Deindividuation is Known as 'The Bystander Effect'[32]

Kitty Genovese highlighted the diffusion of responsibility theory. She was a young woman who was sexually assaulted and brutally murdered at the entrance of her large apartment block. It was reported in the *New York Post* that many witnesses heard her screaming but nobody went to her aid, believing that somebody else would. The facts of this story have since been shown to be inaccurate, but the diffusion of responsibility is still a valid concept.

---

l) Consent in Minors

Gillick Competence

This is used in medical law to determine if a child under the age of 16 is able to consent to his or her own medical treatment without the need for parental consent.

Mrs. Victoria Gillick took her local authority and the department of health to court after she learned that her general practitioner had given contraceptive advise and treatment to her daughter without parental consent.

The case went to the House of Lords, which ruled that:

> the parental right to determine whether or not a minor child below the age of sixteen will have medical treatment terminates if the child achieves sufficient understanding and intelligence to understand fully what is proposed.[33]

The Fraser guidelines deal with the issues of contraception specifically. Gillick competence can be applied to other medical situations.

The Fraser guidelines state that consent is legal where:

- The young person understands the professional's advice.
- The young person cannot be persuaded to inform their parents.
- The young person is likely to begin, or to continue having, sexual intercourse with or without contraceptive treatment.
- Unless the young person receives contraceptive treatment, their physical or mental health, or both, are likely to suffer.
- The young person's best interests require them to receive contraceptive advice or treatment with or without parental consent.[34]

Notes

1. Allport G. W. (1961). *Pattern and Growth in Personality*. Fort Worth, TX: Harcourt College Publisher, p. 28.
2. Weinberg, R. S., and D. Gould. (1999). Personality and Sport. *Foundations of Sport and Exercise Psychology*: 25–46.
3. Freud, S. (1923). The Ego and the Id. *SE*, 19: 1–66.
4. Kassin, S. (2003). *Psychology*. Upper Saddle River, NJ: Prentice-Hall, Inc.
5. Allport, G. W. (1937). *Personality: A Psychological Interpretation*. New York: Holt, Rinehart, & Winston.
6. Cattell, R. B., and H. W. Eber. (1957). *Handbook for the Sixteen Personality Factor Questionnaire*. Champaign, IL: Institute for Personality & Ability Testing.
7. Eysenck, H. J., and S. B. G. Eysenck. (1975). *Manual of the Eysenck Personality Questionnaire*. London: Hodder and Stoughton.
8. Briley, D. A., and E. M. Tucker-Drob. (2014). Genetic and Environmental Continuity in Personality Development: A Meta-Analysis. *Psychological Bulletin*, 140 (5): 1303–1331.
9. Ekman, P., E. R. Sorenson, and W. V. Friesen. (1969). Pan-Cultural Elements in Facial Displays of Emotions. *Science*, 164, 86–88.
10. Lang, P. J. (1994). The Varieties of Emotional Experience: A Meditation on James-Lange Theory. *Psychological Review*, 101 (2): 211–221.
11. Friedman, B. H. (2010). Feelings and the Body: The Jamesian Perspective on Autonomic Specificity of Emotion. *Biological Psychology*, 84: 383–393.
12. Cotton, J. L. (1981). A Review of Research on Schachter's Theory of Emotion and the Misattribution of Arousal. *European Journal of Social Psychology*, 11: 365–397.

13. Smith, C. A., and R. S. Lazarus. (1990). Chapter 23: Emotion and Adaptation. In L. A. Pervin (Ed.), *Handbook of Personality: Theory and Research*. New York: Guilford, pp. 609–637.
14. Maslow, A. H. (1943). A Theory of Human Motivation. *Psychological Review*, 50 (4): 370–396.
15. Fishbein, M., and I. Ajzen. (1975). *Beliefs, Attitude, Intention, and Behavior: An Introduction to Theory and Research*. Reading, MA: Addison-Wesley.
16. Katz, D. (1960). The Functional Approach to the Study of Attitudes. *Public Opinion Quarterly*, 24 (2): 163.
17. Krosnick, J. A., C. M. Judd, and B. Wittenbrink. (2005). The Measurement of Attitudes. In D. Albarracín, B. T. Johnson, and M. P. Zanna (Eds.), *The Handbook of Attitudes*. Mahwah, NJ: Lawrence Erlbaum Associates, pp. 21–76.
18. Horst, P. (1955). L. L. Thurstone and the Science of Human Behavior. *Science*, 122 (3183): 1259–1260.
19. Festinger, L. (1957). *A Theory of Cognitive Dissonance*. Stanford, CA: Stanford University Press.
20. Gallup, G. G. Jr. (1970). Chimpanzees: Self Recognition. *Science*, 167 (3914): 86–87.
21. Premack, D. G., and G. Woodruff. (1978). Does the Chimpanzee Have a Theory of Mind? *Behavioral and Brain Sciences*, 1 (4): 515–526.
22. Baron-Cohen, S., A. M. Leslie, and U. Frith. (1985). Does the Autistic Child Have a "Theory of Mind"? *Cognition*, 21 (1): 37–46.
23. Haney, C., W. C. Banks, and P. G. Zimbardo. (1973). Study of Prisoners and Guards in a Simulated Prison. In *Naval Research Reviews*. Washington, DC: Office of Naval Research, Vol. 9, pp. 1–17.
24. Schuman, S. H., S. Olansky, E. Rivers, C. A. Smith, and D. S. Rambo. (1955). Untreated Syphilis in the Male Negro: Background and Current Status of Patients in the Tuskegee Study. *Journal of Chronic Diseases*, 2 (5): 543–558.
25. Galliher, J. F., W. Brekhus, and D. P. Keys. (2004). *Laud Humphreys: Prophet of Homosexuality and Sociology*. Madison, WI: University of Wisconsin Press.
26. Milgram, S. (1963). Behavioral Study of Obedience. *Journal of Abnormal and Social Psychology*, 67: 371–378.
27. Hevesi, D. (25 September 2010). Robert W. McCollum, Dean of Dartmouth Medical School, Dies at 85. *The New York Times*. [Accessed September 26, 2010].
28. Asch, S. E. (1951). Effects of Group Pressure Upon the Modification and Distortion of Judgment. In H. Guetzkow (Ed.), *Groups, Leadership and Men*. Pittsburgh, PA: Carnegie Press.
29. Rioch, M. J. (1970). The Work of Wilfred Bion on Groups. *Psychiatry*, 33 (1), 56–66.
30. Janis, I. L. (1972). *Victims of Groupthink: A Psychological Study of Foreign-Policy Decisions and Fiascoes*. Boston: Houghton Mifflin.
31. Smith, M. B., and L. Mann. (1992, June). Irving L. Janis (1918–1990): Obituary. *American Psychologist*, 47 (6): 812–813.
32. Darley, J. M., and B. Latane. (1968). Bystander Intervention in Emergencies: Diffusion of Responsibility. *Journal of Personality and Social Psychology*, 8 (4p1): 377.
33. Gillick v West Norfolk and Wisbech AHA [1985] UKHL 7. British and Irish Legal Information Institute. [Accessed February 19, 2017].
34. Cornock, M. (2007, July). Fraser Guidelines or Gillick Competence? *Journal of Children's and Young People's Nursing*, 1 (3): 142–142.

3 Sociocultural Psychiatry

Elizabeth Templeton

a) Ethics

There are three distinct ethical principles that should be understood:

Teleological systems focus on *consequences*: 'the rightness of an act is determined by its end', so the emphasis is on the consequence of an action. This might be referred to as 'consequentialism'. *Utilitarianism* is an example of this.

Deontological ethics place an emphasis on *a person's action* rather than their consequence. The morality of an action can be determined if a person has breached an obligation/rule or duty. You may hear to this being referred to as *rule-based ethics*.

Virtue-based ethics, where the emphasis is on *moral character* and the reasoning behind an action.

Text Box 3.1

Virtue ethics and Utilitarianism

Virtue is generally agreed to be a character trait, and the ethical principle emphasises the moral character of an individual as the driving force for an ethical behaviour. Virtue ethics can also be referred to as *eudaimonism*, a state of happiness, and—in the context of virtue ethics—'human flourishing'.

Utilitarianism is a moral principle that holds that the morally right course of action in any situation is the one that produces the greatest balance of benefits over harms for everyone affected.

The ethical principles in Table 3.1 are commonly applied to health care and should be understood for membership exams.

DOI: 10.1201/9781003322573-5

Table 3.1 Basic ethical principles

Basic ethical principles
Autonomy—a patient's right to choose and make decisions regarding the care they receive.
Beneficence—a doctor should always act in a way that benefits the patient.
Non-maleficence—a doctor should never act in a way that will cause harm to the patient.
Justice—all patients will be treated equally and fairly.

According to W. D. **Ross**, there are several *prima facie duties* that we should apply when making decisions, which include:

* Fidelity
* Reparation (duty to make up harm done to others)
* Gratitude
* Non-injury
* Harm-prevention

b) Global Ethical Policies

Declaration of Geneva (Physician's Oath) declares a doctor's dedication to the *humanitarian goals* of medicine. It was introduced following the Nazi doctors' trial in Nuremberg.

Declaration of Helsinki outlines *ethical principles* regarding human experimentation.

Declaration of Tokyo states that doctors should not participate or condone the act of *torture* or cruel treatment of prisoners.

Declaration of Lisbon outlines the principal *rights of the patients* that the medical profession endorses.

Declaration of Ottawa launched a series of actions among international organisations to achieve the goal of '*health for all*'.

Text Box 3.2

Social Class

Social class 0	Unemployed or student
Social class I	Professional
Social class II	Intermediate
Social class III	Skilled, manual, or clerical
Social class IV	Semi-skilled
Social class V	Unskilled

c) Human Rights

The Human Rights Act became law in 1998 and incorporated the rights contained in the European Convention on Human Rights into UK law.

Human rights are 'rights and freedoms to which all humans are entitled'. These are:

1. The right to *life*.
2. Freedom from *torture* and degrading treatment.
3. Freedom from *slavery* and forced labour.
4. The right to *liberty*.
5. The right to a *fair trial*.
6. The right not to be *punished* for something that wasn't a crime when you did it.
7. The right to respect for *private* and family life.
8. Freedom of *thought, conscience and religion* and freedom to express your beliefs.
9. Freedom of *expression*.
10. Freedom of *assembly and association*.
11. The right to *marry* and to start a *family*.
12. The right not to be *discriminated* against in respect of these rights and freedoms.
13. The right to *peaceful* enjoyment of your property.
14. The right to an *education*.

d) Models of Illness

International classifications of impairments, disabilities and handicaps provide a conceptual framework of the consequences of illness:

*   **Impairment**—the structural or psychological *damage* to the person, for example, a broken leg.
*   **Disability**—the *inability to carry out activities* of daily living as a result of the impairment, for example, unable to stand and prepare food.
*   **Handicap**—the *social disadvantage* resulting from the disability, for example, time of work.

The 'Sick Role'

Described by American sociologist Talcott **Parsons**:

*   The sick person is exempt from carrying out normal social roles.
*   The sick person is not blamed or directly responsible for their illness.
*   The sick person should make appropriate attempts to seek medical attention or get better.
*   Disease refers to the pathology of an illness.

- Illness refers to the personal experience of feeling ill.
- Sickness refers to the social consequences of being unwell.[1]

Health Belief Model

This was first developed in the 1950s by social psychologists Godfrey H. **Hochbaum,** Irwin **Rosenstock** and Stephen **Kegeles** working in the US public health services.

They used the attitudes and experiences of individuals to help explain and predict health behaviours.

The model identifies several patient beliefs that might impact their treatment participation:

Core Beliefs

- Belief about the severity of their illness.
- Belief about the susceptibility of acquiring the disease or complications.
- Belief about the direct financial cost of treatment and indirect costs to the person's time and effort.
- Belief about the benefit or success of treatment.
- Beliefs regarding the environment and social cues to accept the treatment.

The Transtheoretical Model (TTM)

Developed by James **Prochaska** and Carlo **DiClemente** (1982),[2] this model aims to describe how a person can change their behaviour or acquire a new behaviour.

They identified five key methods that encourage a person to change their behaviour:

- **Autonomy**—increasing awareness of alternative treatments/behaviours.
- **Increasing awareness** of the problem and its consequences—for example, a smoker learning about lung cancer.
- **Catharsis**—emotional acknowledgement of the problem and the process of change.
- **Conditional stimuli**—involves *counter conditioning*: developing an alternative behaviour and avoidance of stimuli associated with the behaviour, for example, a patient who smokes might avoid situations he might smoke in or replace the smoking behaviour so that every time he has a drink, he chews gum afterwards instead of smoking.
- **Positive reinforcement**—from others and self-reinforcement.

From these processes, Prochaska and DiClemente developed five stages of change:

- **Precontemplation**—the person has not yet considered changing their behaviour and does not see it as a problem.

- **Contemplation**—the person starts to consider changing their behaviour and becomes more aware of the pros and cons of doing this. A person can stay in this stage for a long time if they see the pros and cons as equal; for example, 'if I give up smoking, I will have more money, but I also won't enjoy my nights out as much'.
- **Preparation**—the person develops plans to change the behaviour; for example, they tell friends they are going to quit smoking, throwing away any cigarettes in the house.
- **Action**—the person carries out the behavioural change: the person stops smoking.
- **Maintenance**—the person maintains the behavioural change.

e) Family Life

General systems model of families regards each family member as connected emotionally and each action of the family produces a reciprocal reaction in one of its members and vice versa.

This is *the basis of family therapy.*

Theodore **Lidz**[3] was an advocate for *environmental causes of schizophrenia,* believing too much emphasis was placed on the biological causes. He researched family life in relation to schizophrenia and proposed two 'shizophrenogenic' patterns:

- **Marital skew**—the family will often be calm and harmonious; for example, one parent might be dominant in their views about how to raise a child, whilst the other might be submissive. Therefore, the unchallenged psychotic or bizarre beliefs by the dominant parents become reality for the family.
- **Marital schism**—this family is in a state of disequilibrium due to parental discord, where parents are often near the point of separation and may collude with the child and belittle the parental ability of the other.

Causal links between family members and schizophrenia are widely disputed due to the lack of robust research, and this line of thinking of has fallen out of favour in contemporary times.

f) Theory of Expressed Emotion (EE)

Developed by George **Brown** and Michael **Rutter**,[4] this theory looked at how the family of a schizophrenic patient will talk spontaneously about the patient.

The degree of EE within a family is determined by the *Camberwell family interview*, a structured interview that takes into account five measures:

- Positive remarks
- Critical remarks
- Emotional warmth

- Hostility
- Over involvement

Interviewers also took into account the views of the patient in regard to their parents.

This research has shown that patients living in high EE families are *more likely to relapse* than patients who do not live in high EE families.

g) Society and Mental Health

George **Engel's BioPsychoSocial model** is widely used by psychiatrists in aetiological formulations.

Social causation theory—proposes that mental illness is caused by lower social class and poverty. This theory does not hold true for conditions such as bipolar affective disorder and schizophrenia.

Social drift theory—recognises that whilst schizophrenic patients are over-represented in social class V, their parents are not. This implies that mental illness results in a downward drift of economic status.

Social construction theory—proposes that mental illness has been constructed by certain groups in society (for example, doctors, lawyers or politicians) for their own personal interests.

For example, agoraphobia might reflect historical sexism against women that prevented them from using public spaces safely.

Text Box 3.3

The Great Smoky Mountains Study[5]

This study looked at the *effect of poverty* on psychopathology.

The participants were American and Native American children, assessed within groups of 'poor families', 'never poor families' and 'ex-poor families'.

The 'ex-poor' families lived in an area that had been given an increased income after the building of a large casino on Native American land.

The study demonstrated that after the casino opened, the rates of psychiatric issues between the 'ex-poor' fell and were equal to that of the 'never poor'.

The conditions most likely to respond to reducing poverty were oppositional defiant disorder and conduct disorders.

---

h) History of Major Publications in Psychiatry

Table 3.2 provides a list of historically significant publications in psychiatry.

Table 3.2 History of major publications in psychiatry

Michel Foucault	*Madness and Civilization*
Ronald Laing	*The Divided Self*
Sigmund Freud	*The Interpretation of Dreams* 'Beyond the Pleasure Principle' *The Psychopathology of Everyday Life*
Thomas Szasz	*The Myth of Mental Illness*
Erving Goffman	*Asylums* *The Presentation of Self in Everyday Life* Goffman is credited with coining the word *stigma* and worked extensively in this area.
Émile Durkheim	*Le suicide*
Tom Main	*The Ailment*
Jerome Frank	*Persuasion and Healing*
George Brown and Tirril Harris	'Social Origins of Depression'
Ugo Cerletti	Associated with electroconvulsive therapy (ECT)
Egas Moniz	Associated with frontal leucotomy

i) Important Figures in Psychiatry

It is important to remember who coined the following well known psychological terms, as these often come up in membership exams:

- **Donald Winnicott**—good enough mother, transitional object.
- **Carl Jung**—collective unconscious, archetype, anima, animus.
- **Melanie Klein**—paranoid-schizoid position, depressive position, splitting.
- **Sigmund Freud**—free association, transference, Ego, Superego, Ed, *Eros*, Thanatos, defence mechanisms, Oedipus complex, the unconscious.
- **Wilfred Bion**—basic assumptions group.
- **Kurt Lewin**—group dynamics.
- **Jacob L. Moreno**—group psychotherapy.
- **Karen Horney**—womb envy.
- **Erving Goffman**—total institution.
- **Siegfried Foulkes**—foundation matrix.
- **Russell Barton**—institutional neurosis.
- **Bénédict Morel**—demence precoce (1852). Not clearly used to describe a specific schizophrenia syndrome.
- **Emil Kraepelin**—dementia Praecox (1893) and manic depression.
- **Ewald Hecker**—hebephrenia.

- **Karl Ludwig Kahlbaum**—catatonia.
- **Eugen Bleuler**—schizophrenia.
- **Jacob Kasanin**—schizoaffective.
- **George Miller Beard**—neurasthenia.
- **Karl Kleist**—unipolar and bipolar.
- **James Braid**—hypnosis.
- **Julius Ludwig August Koch**—psychopathic inferiority.
- **Johann Christian Reil**—psychiatry.

j) Immigration and Schizophrenia

Schizophrenia is seen more frequently in migrant populations than native populations. This phenomenon is also observed in other mental disorders, but schizophrenia is the most researched.

The following list summarises the main findings:

The incidence of schizophrenia appears to be *higher in second generation Afro-Caribbean immigrants* than in first generation immigrants; furthermore, *incidence rates of schizophrenia in Caribbean countries appear similar to those seen in the indigenous UK population.* This implies that the change in environment—rather than genetics—plays a significant role.

A concept of pre-psychotic segregation has been proposed, stating that people with schizophrenia find it hard to live in their countries of birth and might be more likely to emigrate. However, the later finding that rates are higher in second generation immigrants means that this is an unlikely explanation.

The increased rate of schizophrenia is seen among Afro-Caribbean, African and—to a lesser degree—Asian immigrants, so *the explanation cannot be purely biological or race specific.*

The study Aetiology & Ethnicity in Schizophrenia and other Psychosis[6] **(AESOP)**, conducted in London, Bristol and Nottingham, found that:

Afro-Caribbeans had a ninefold increase in the rates of psychosis.

Ethnic minorities were much more likely to be detained in psychiatric hospitals using sections of the Mental Health Act, and also accessed help more frequently through the police than through their general practitioners.

London had a twofold rate of psychosis compared to the other two centres.

k) Stigma

Stigma is an *attribute or trait considered to be shameful* that sets a person apart as inferior or unacceptable. Types of stigma are explained in Table 3.3.

'Changing Minds' was a five-year campaign designed by the Royal College of Psychiatrists in response to an earlier survey which showed 70% of people believed that people with schizophrenia are violent and unpredictable. The campaign created several innovative media projects aimed at tackling mental health stigma. One of the better known was called *1 in 4*, a short film

Table 3.3 Types of Stigma

Types of stigma:	
Felt stigma	Refers to a person's *fear of stigma*; it is considered *more disabling* than enacted stigma.
Enacted stigma	A person's *experience of discrimination*.
Self-stigma	A prejudice that person might hold *about themselves*; this internalised stigma develops as a result of societal views.
Public stigma	The negative *reaction of the general population* to a specific trait or attribute.
Courtesy stigma	Refers to the stigma experienced by a person with a *close association* to a person who bears a stigma.

that aimed to challenge preconceptions about mental health; the title highlights how common mental health problems are.

l) Grief

Grief Reaction

John **Bowlby** described the stages of grief. He observed that people can go back and forth between the stages and that there is no specific time frame to move from one to another.

- **Shock and disbelief**—first few days.
- **Yearning and anger**—first few weeks.
- **Despair and acceptance of loss**—several months.
- **Resolution**—1–2 years.

The **Kubler-Ross** model of grief stages can be remembered as **DABDA**:

  Denial > Anger > Bargaining > Depression > Acceptance

Abnormal Grief

Some people might experience a *delayed grief reaction*, in which there is a marked lack of grief symptoms in the first two weeks as they consciously or subconsciously make an effort to avoid painful emotions.

  Other might experience a *prolonged grief reaction* and demonstrate grief related symptoms long after death (>6 months).

  Features of abnormal grief:

- **Generalised guilt**—not just specifically related to the deceased
- **Suicidal thoughts**
- **Hallucinations**—not of the deceased
- **Feelings of worthlessness**

Notes

1. Parsons, T. (1975, Summer). The Sick Role and the Role of the Physician Reconsidered. *Millbank Memorial Fund Quarterly*, 53 (3): 257–278.
2. Prochaska, J. O., and C. C. DiClemente. (1982). Transtheoretical Therapy: Toward a More Integrative Model of Change. *Psychotherapy: Theory, Research & Practice*, 19 (3): 276–288.
3. Lidz, R. W., and T. Lidz. (1949). The Family Environment of Schizophrenic Patients. *American Journal of Psychiatry*, 106: 332–345.
4. Brown, G. W., and M. Rutter. (1966). The Measurement of Family Activities and Relationships: A Methodological Study. *Human Relations*, 19: 241–258.
5. Copeland, W., L. Shanahan, E. J. Costello, and A. Angold. (2011). Cumulative Prevalence of Psychiatric Disorders by Young Adulthood: A Prospective Cohort Analysis From the Great Smoky Mountains Study. *Journal of the American Academy of Child & Adolescent Psychiatry*, 50 (3): 252–261.
6. Fearon, P., J. B. Kirkbride, C. Morgan, P. Dazzan, K. Morgan, T. Lloyd, . . . R. Mallett. (2006). Incidence of Schizophrenia and Other Psychoses in Ethnic Minority Groups: Results from the MRC AESOP Study. *Psychological Medicine*, 36 (11): 1541–1550.

Part II
Human Development

4 Theories of Human Development

Richard Kerslake

a) Piaget's Theory of Cognitive Development[1]

Jean Piaget (1896–1980) theorised that a child's thinking develops through ordered stages (Table 4.1) involving 'schemas': building blocks of knowledge which provide structure to understanding the world and organising past experiences to provide a model that can be referenced in the future.

Children will combine and integrate schemas via organisation in order to be able to adjust to a new situation and achieve adaptation.

Adaptation: how children progress through Piaget's stages of development. This is achieved through:

Assimilation: new experiences are understood through existing schemas to reach 'equilibrium',

and

Accommodation: existing schemas are changed when new experiences result in 'disequilibrium'.

N.B., Accommodation will change a new schema; in assimilation the schema will stay the same.

Sensorimotor Stage

During the sensorimotor stage, children are coordinating sensory inputs and motor capabilities into schema that allow them to manipulate their environment and using reflex activity of innate reflexes (grasping, sucking, looking) to understand the external world.

Primary circular reactions trial coordination of reflexes to stimulate *own body* and senses, for example, making sounds.
Secondary circular reactions seek to stimulate response *outside own body*, for example, shaking a rattle.

DOI: 10.1201/9781003322573-7

Table 4.1 Piaget's stages

0–2 years	Sensorimotor stage
2–7 years	Pre-operational stage
7–11 years	Concrete operational stage
11—end of adolescence	Formal operational stage

Tertiary circular reactions seek to produces novel behaviours through curiosity and experimentation, for example, dropping spoon on the floor.

Object permanence develops during the sensorimotor stage at 18–24 months: objects exist when they are no longer visible.

Preoperational Stage

Language and symbolic thinking begins. Logic has NOT developed.

Animistic thinking: attributing *life-like qualities* to inanimate objects, for example, 'Teddy is hungry'.

Transductive reasoning: assuming separate concrete events that happen together are *causally linked*, for example, thunder causes rain (deductive and inductive reasoning occur in adolescence).

Semiotic function: a symbol can *represent* something, for example, a stick drawing represents a person.

Egocentrism: refers to being unable to interpret the world from the *perspective of other*, demonstrated by Piaget's three mountain experiment.

Box 4.1

Piaget's Three Mountain Experiment

Scenario: three mountains are positioned in a triangle with the child asked to describe the view of a person standing on each mountain (Figure 4.1).

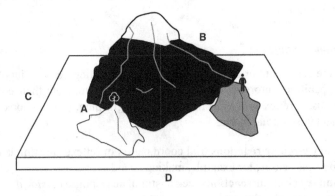

Figure 4.1 Three mountain experiment

> Egocentric children assume that other people will see the same view of the three mountains regardless of where they stand.

Concrete Operational Stage

Mastery of mental operations leads to less rigid and more logical thought processes but is still based on real 'concrete' concepts. Abstract thought has NOT developed.

Conservation: understanding that substances are maintained or 'conserved' regardless of the shape or form it is presented, for example, pastry is unchanged when rolled from a ball into a ribbon.
Classification: ability to group items as having various properties with which it can be identified, for example, shape and colour.
Syllogistic reasoning: a logical conclusion is formed from the premises.
Reversibility: understanding that substances can change between forms, for example, ice to water and back again.
Loss of egocentric thought: enables children to consider someone else's perspective.

Formal Operational Stage

Development of abstract thinking and testing hypotheses begins. Thinking is idealistic, about how the world 'ought to be'.

Deductive reasoning: applies general concepts to a particular matter.

b) The Zone of Proximal Development

Lev **Vygotsky** (1978)[2] proposed a more *social context* to child development describing the *zone of proximal development*, being the difference between the child's current developmental capacity and that which is attainable with appropriate assistance.

c) Kohlberg's Theory of Moral Development

Lawrence **Kohlberg** (1984)[3] proposed that human *morality*, knowing right from wrong, is learned in stages (Figure 4.2). N.B., this doesn't necessarily equate to morally correct behaviour!

This theory was developed after a study on 72 males aged 10–16 years who were presented with dilemma tests such as the 'Heinz dilemma'.

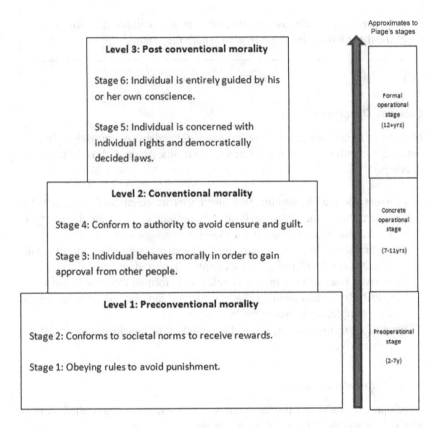

Figure 4.2 Kohlberg's theory of moral development

d) Freud's Stages of Psychosexual Development (1905)[4]

So-called because each stage represents the fixation of *sexual instincts* on different parts of the body.

Each stage, outlined in Table 4.2, requires resolution of a *conflict* before progressing to the next stage, requiring the expenditure of *libido*.

e) Erikson's Stages of Psychosocial Development[5]

Erik **Erikson** (1959) proposed eight stages extending from infancy through adulthood. These stages correspond with a specific 'crisis' contributing to how personality is developed.

Erikson's model was influenced by Freud, but Erikson focussed on the role of *culture and society* as creating conflict. As these become resolved, a 'basic virtue' is established and so the ego develops.

Table 4.2 Freud's Stages of Psychosexual Development

Aide memoire: Old Age Pensioners Love Grapes	Oral:	Mouth	Understanding the world through sucking, biting, swallowing. *Ego develops.*
	Anal:	Anus	Understanding the world through expelling or retaining of bowel or bladder.
	Phallic:	Penis or clitoris	Males pass through Oedipal complex. Females pass through the Electra complex. *Superego develops.*
	Latent:		Little libido present.
	Genital:	Penis or vagina	Sexual intercourse.

0–18 Months

Trust vs. Mistrust: understanding the world is generally safe, despite the potential for fear and unpredictability.

  Basic virtue = Hope

18–36 Months

Autonomy vs. Shame: learning to be independent whilst tolerating failure.

  Basic virtue = Will

36 Months–7 Years

Initiative vs. Guilt: developing capacity as planners and leaders, without being oversensitive to criticism.

  Basic virtue = Purpose

7–12 Years

Industry vs. Inferiority: having confidence in personal strengths rather than doubting one's potential.

  Basic virtue = Competence

12–18 Years

Identity vs. Role Confusion: understanding one's identity and developing a sense of self.

  Basic virtue = Fidelity

18–40 Years

Intimacy vs. Isolation: exploration of, and development of capacity to form, meaningful relationships.

  Basic virtue = Love

40–65 Years

Generativity vs. Stagnation: embedding lifestyle habits and establishing responsibilities to the wider community.
  Basic virtue = Care

65 and Onwards

Integrity vs. Despair: reflecting and contemplating the life lived.
  Basic virtue = Wisdom

f) Mahler's 'Separation-Individuation' Stages of Child Development (1968)[6]

Table 4.3 Mahler's Stages of Child Development

Autistic phase	In the first few weeks of life, the child is mostly sleeping, cut off and self-absorbed.
Symbiotic phase	Up to 5 months, the child is aware of the mother but doesn't consider itself separate.
Separation-individuation phase	Child differentiates itself from the mother and develops in own identity through sub-phases: hatching, practising and reproachment.

g) Table of Relevant Developmental Stages

Table 4.4 Developmental stage theories.

	0–2 years		2–7 years	7–12 years	13+ years
Piaget	Sensorimotor		Pre-operational	Concrete operational	Formal operational
Kohlberg			Pre-conventional morality	Conventional morality	Post-conventional morality
	0–18 months	**18–36 months**	**3–7 years**	**7–12 years**	**13+ years**
Freud	Oral	Anal	Phallic	Latency	Genital
Erikson	Trust vs. mistrust	Autonomy vs. shame	Initiative vs. guilt	Industry vs. inferiority	Identity vs. role confusion

h) Temperament

Arnold **Buss** and Robert **Plomin** (1984)[7] described temperament as 'traits observable by two years of age that are genetic in origin'. These were conceptualised as *E*motionality, *A*ctivity and *S*ociability and were thought to predict adult personality, whereas *character* was proposed as a result of *learned* experiences.

Alexander **Thomas** and Stella **Chess** (1968),[8] in their New York Longitudinal Study, used factor analysis to categorise nine temperamental features into three clusters:

- 'Easy child'—40%
- 'Difficult child'—10%
- 'Slow to warm up child'—15%
- Does not fall into a category—35%

i) Fear

Specific fears are thought to have a developmental trend which correspond with age (Table 4.5).

Table 4.5 Ages associated with specific fears

0–6 months	Falling and sensory overload, for example, loud noises
6–12 months	Heights
1 year	Separation, strangers
2–3 years	Darkness, animals
5–8 years	Monsters
9–12 years	Injury, disasters
Adolescence	Social criticism

j) Speech/Language Milestones

Ages associated with language development are outlined in Table 4.6.

Table 4.6 Ages associated with usual language development

6 months	Babbling, laughing/crying
1 year	Single words
2 years	Two consecutive words, vocab of 5–20 words (nouns > verbs)
3 years	Three consecutive words, counts to ten
4 years	Vocab up to 1,000 words, use of plurals and tenses
5 years	Adult-like speech

Risk factors associated with delayed speech:[9]

- Family history of speech and language delay
- Male gender
- Perinatal factors, for example, twins
- Educational levels of parents
- Childhood illnesses
- Birth order
- Family size

k) Motor Milestones

Ages associated with motor milestones are outlined in Table 4.7.

Table 4.7 Motor milestones

Age	Motor milestone
Birth	Mostly sleeps
4 weeks	Responds to movement or noise.
6 weeks	First smile.
3 months	Holds head up unaided.
6 months	Sitting unaided, rolls from front to back.
12 months	Cruising by holding furniture.
18 months	Walking independently.
24–30 months	Climbing/descending stairs unaided with rails, running.
3 years	Feeding and simple dressing oneself.
4 years	Hops on one leg.
5 years	Climbing/descending stairs one foot at a time.

Table 4.8 Copying shapes

3 years	Circle
4 years	Cross
4½ years	Square
5 years	Triangle
7 years	Diamond

l) Attachment Theory

Developed by John **Bowlby** (1969),[10] attachment theory describes the *innate* tendency to form *emotional bonds* between persons, in particular between mother and child, thought to *improve survival* chances. Bowlby focussed on the *primary caregiver* as the *principal attachment figure*, identified by the infant in the *first three months*.

Monotropy describes the preference for a single caregiver.

Subsidiary attachments could be formed.

Attachment concepts:

Proximity seeking to the attachment figure, especially when frightened.

A **secure base** is ideally provided by the primary caregiver, within which the infant can safely explore its environment.

Separation anxiety when distanced from primary caregiver, around *10–18 months*, usually diminished at 4 years.

A positive response to strangers is seen between 14–18 weeks, replaced by **stranger anxiety** around *8 months*.

The **critical period** of attachment is between *6–36 months*, when the infant is vulnerable to interruptions in attachments.

A lack of secure early life attachments was proposed as a predictor of difficulty forming close relationships in adulthood.

Attachment is a *dyadic interdependent relationship*, not the fault of infant or caregiver.

Attachment behaviour is usually stable over a lifetime.

A child will develop an *internal working model* to understand future relationships. This is a cognitive framework, organised within the psyche of the child.

Poorly developed attachments are related to psychopathology later in life but are *not causative* for specific psychiatric disorders of adulthood.

Intergenerational transmission of poorly developed attachments has been demonstrated, that is, children with poorly developed attachments will struggle to develop stable attachments with their own children.

m) Studies Related to Attachment

Konrad **Lorenz**'s (1935) *imprinting* theory[11] proposed that geese identify their mother as the first moving object they see, during a *12–17-hour critical period* after hatching. The experiment involved hatching a clutch of goose eggs, half under a goose mother, half beside himself. When the geese hatched beside him, the young birds regarded him as their mother and followed him accordingly. The other group followed the mother goose.

John **Dollard** and Neal **Miller**'s (1950) behavioural theory[12] stated that the infants will initially form an attachment to whoever feeds it, through the process of *classical conditioning*, learned behaviours.

Harry **Harlow** (1958)[13] studied newborn rhesus monkeys bonding with mothers. He contradicted the behavioural theories by demonstrating that mothers providing 'tactile comfort' became an attachment figure in preference to mothers providing food.

Rudolph **Schaffer** and Peggy **Emerson** (1964)[14] studied 60 babies at monthly intervals for the first 18 months of life.

Three measures were recorded:

- **Stranger anxiety**—response to arrival of a stranger.
- **Separation anxiety**—distress level when separated from carer; degree of comfort needed on return.
- **Social referencing**—degree that child looks at carer to check how they should respond to something new (secure base).

This demonstrated that infant attachments develop in the following sequence:

(0–6 weeks) **Asocial**: social and non-social stimuli produce a favourable reaction, such as a smile.

(6 weeks to 7 months) **Indiscriminate attachments**: indiscriminate enjoyment of human company, regardless of the caregiver.

From 3 months, infants smile more at familiar faces and can be easily comforted by a regular caregiver.

(7–9 months) **Specific attachment**: preference develops for a single attachment figure for comfort and reassurance. Stranger fear and separation anxiety first noted, seen as evidence that the baby has formed an attachment.

(10 months and onwards) **Multiple attachments**: infants become more independent to form several attachments.

The **National Institute of Child Health and Human Development Study**,[15] started in 1991, found no significant effects on the attachments of children attending day care within the first year of their life.

n) Mary Ainsworth (1973)[16]

Mary **Ainsworth** collaborated with Bowlby to demonstrate differences in the quality of attachments, by using the *Strange Situation Procedure*. The behaviour of a 12–18-month-old child is observed during eight episodes:

* Mother, baby and experimenter (lasts less than one minute)
* Mother and baby alone
* A stranger joins mother and infant
* Mother leaves baby and stranger alone to interact
* Mother returns (reunion behaviour noted) and stranger leaves
* Mother leaves and infant left completely alone (separation protest noted)
* Stranger returns (stranger anxiety noted)
* Mother returns and stranger leaves (reunion behaviour noted)

The experimenter observes for five primary interaction behaviours:

* Proximity and contacting seeking
* Contact maintaining
* Avoidance of proximity and contact
* Resistance to contact and comforting
* Searching

Ainsworth identified three main *childhood attachment* styles: secure, insecure avoidant and insecure ambivalent/resistant.

Mary **Main** developed the *Adult Attachment Interview* (AAI), a semi structured interview to establish an *adult's attachment* to their parents, classified as either 'secure', 'dismissing', 'preoccupied' or 'disorganised' (Table 4.9).

Mary **Main** and Judith **Solomon** (1986)[17] identified a fourth attachment style where behaviour was *disorganised* in the presence of the primary caregiver.

Table 4.9 Main's attachment styles

	Secure attachment	Ambivalent/resistant attachment	Insecure/avoidant attachment
Separation anxiety	Distressed when mother leaves.	Infant distressed when mother leaves.	Infant shows no sign of distress when mother leaves.
Stranger anxiety	Avoids the stranger when alone, but friendly when mother is present.	Infant is fearful and avoids the stranger.	Infant appears unaffected when the stranger is present and plays normally.
Reunion behaviour	Positive and happy when mother returns.	Infant approaches mother but resists contact, sometimes pushing her away.	Infant shows disinterest when mother returns.
Other	Mother used as a safe base to explore the environment.	Infant cries more and explores less than the other two types.	Mother and stranger are equally able to comfort the infant.
% of infants	70	15	15

This is often seen in children who have experienced early life *abuse* and *neglect.*

N.B., whilst insecure attachments are more common where there is mental illness in the relationship between the child and caregiver, many such relationships do form secure attachments.

o) Developmental Concepts

Heinz **Wimmer** and Josef **Perner** (1983)[18] described *theory of mind*, an individual's ability to consider the thoughts and motivations of others. This is demonstrated through 'false belief tasks' such as the *Sally and Anne* test. Theory of mind usually develops around *age 4* but is shown to be lacking where autistic spectrum disorder is diagnosed.

Gender identity is thought to develop around age 3.

However, acting in *gender roles* is thought to develop through social conditioning.

p) Parenting Styles

Diana Baumrind (1966)[19] studied preschool children to identify different styles of parenting (Table 4.10).

q) Freudian Concepts

Aggression was explained as a result of a primary *death instinct*, which was named *Thanatos*, an urge in each of us to cause destruction.

Table 4.10 Parenting styles

Authoritative parenting	• Child's activities are directed but with reasoning and flexibility • Nurturing approach rather than punishing	• Confident and capable, happy disposition • Able to emotionally regulate
Authoritarian parenting	• Imposing strict rules • Values obedience • Forceful measures to curb self-will	• Anxious and withdrawn • Obedient and proficient • Poor tolerance of frustration
Permissive parenting	• Accepting approach • Rare discipline • Avoid confrontation with the child	• Tends towards poor emotional regulation • Problems with authority • See themselves as unhappy

Freud also described an opposing *life instinct* called *Eros*.

Catharsis was described as the process of *discharging libidinal energy*, by performing or watching an aggressive act, in order to feel calmer.

The **topographical model of the mind** divided the mind into three regions:

- The **conscious** system, where one is *aware*.
- The **preconscious** system, where there isn't awareness of information, but it could *easily be brought into the conscious* system.
- The **unconscious** system, *outside of conscious* awareness. This operates on *primary process thinking* (aimed at *wish fulfilment*), which is governed by the *pleasure principle* and is *irrational*, allowing for contradictions.

r) Assessment of Intelligence

Various tools are developed to assess a person's *innate cognitive ability* and the capacity to apply it.

The originally calculated for intelligence quotient (IQ) was:

$$\left(IQ\right) = \frac{\text{Mental age}}{\text{Chronological age}} \times 100$$

This calculation was used in the **Stanford-Binet Intelligence Scale**. It uses knowledge, quantitative reasoning, visual-spatial processing, working memory and fluid reasoning. It is criticised for having cultural bias towards different social classes and races. As it was designed for children, the formula implies that IQ declines in old age.

IQ is normally distributed (Figure 4.3) within the population, with 100 being the average.

The Wechsler Adult Intelligence Scale (WAIS) uses age related approximations to provide a 'deviational IQ'. It has three scores: verbal IQ, performance IQ and total IQ (Figure 4.4).

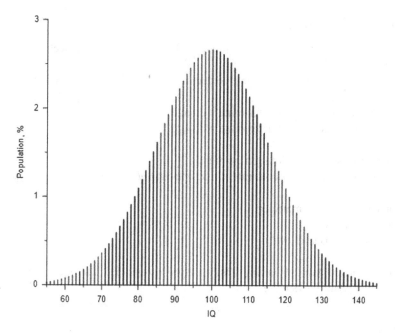

Figure 4.3 IQ distribution

Source: Alessio Damato, Mikhail Ryazanov, CC BY-SA 3.0 <http://creativecommons.org/licenses/by-sa/3.0/>, via Wikimedia Commons

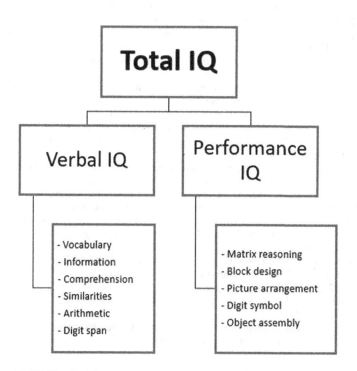

Figure 4.4 WAIS subsections

A difference in verbal: performance IQ of > *15* might indicate *organic involvement*.

The WAIS can indicate cognitive decline using specific components:

- 'Hold tests' = don't deteriorate with age
- 'Don't hold tests' = deteriorate with age

These provide a 'deterioration quotient'.

Where a language or cultural barrier, *non-verbal intelligence tests* are used:

Raven progressive matrices
Draw-a-man test
Seguin-Form Board test

The **National Adult Reading Test** measures *premorbid intelligence* if there has been cognitive decline.

Notes

1. Piaget, J. (1936). *Origins of Intelligence in the Child*. London: Routledge & Kegan Paul.
2. Vygotsky, L. S. (1978). *Mind in Society: The Development of Higher Psychological Processes*. Cambridge, MA: Harvard University Press.
3. Kohlberg, L. (1984). *The Psychology of Moral Development: The Nature and Validity of Moral Stages* (Essays on Moral Development, Volume 2). San Francisco: Harper & Row.
4. Freud, S. (1949). *Three Essays on the Theory of Sexuality*. Oxford: Imago Publ. Co.
5. Erikson, E. H., I. H. Paul, F. Heider, and R. W. Gardner. (1959). Psychological Issues. *International Universities Press*, 1.
6. Mahler, M. S. (1968). *On Human Symbiosis and the Vicissitudes of Individuation. Infantile Psychosis*, Volume 1. New York: International Universities Press.
7. Buss, A., and R. Plomin. (1984). *Temperament: Early Developing Personality Traits*. Hillsdale, NJ: Erlbaum.
8. Thomas, A., S. Chess, and S. G. Birch. (1968). *Temperament and Behaviour Disorders in Children*. New York: New York University Press.
9. Nelson, H. D., P. Nygren, M. Walker, and R. Panoscha. (2006). Screening for Speech and Language Delay in Preschool Children: Systematic Evidence Review for the US Preventive Services Task Force. *Pediatrics*, 117 (2): e298–e319.
10. Bowlby, J. (1969). *Attachment: Attachment and Loss: Vol. 1. Loss*. New York: Basic Books.
11. Lorenz, K. (1935). Der Kumpan in der Umwelt des Vogels: Der Artgenosse als auslösendes Moment sozialer Verhaltensweisen. *Journal für Ornithologie*, 83: 137–215, 289–413.
12. Dollard, J., and N. E. Miller. (1950). *Personality and Psychotherapy*. New York: McGraw-Hill.
13. Harlow, H. F., and R. R. Zimmermann. (1958). The Development of Affective Responsiveness in Infant Monkeys. *Proceedings of the American Philosophical Society*, 102: 501–509.

14. Schaffer, H. R., and P. E. Emerson. (1964). The Development of Social Attachments in Infancy. *Monographs of the Society for Research in Child Development,* 1–77.

15. NICHD Early Child Care Research Network. (2001). Child Care and Family Predictors of Preschool Attachment and Stability from Infancy. *Developmental Psychology*, 37: 847–862.

16. Ainsworth, M. D. S. (1973). The Development of Infant-Mother Attachment. In B. Cardwell and H. Ricciuti (Eds.), *Review of Child Development Research*. Chicago: University of Chicago Press, Vol. 3, pp. 1–94.

17. Main, M., and J. Solomon. (1986). Discovery of a New, Insecure-Disorganized/Disoriented Attachment Pattern. In M. Yogman and T. B. Brazelton (Eds.), *Affective Development in Infancy*. Norwood, NJ: Ablex, pp. 95–124.

18. Wimmer, H., and J. Perner. (1983). Beliefs About Beliefs: Representation and Constraining Function of Wrong Beliefs in Young Children's Understanding of Deception. *Cognition*, 13: 103–128.

19. Baumrind, D. (1966). Effects of Authoritative Parental Control on Child Behavior. *Child Development*, 37 (4): 887–907.

Part III
Basic Neurosciences

5   Neuroanatomy

Elizabeth Templeton

a) Brain Development

The embryonic brain is divided as in Table 5.1.

In the human embryo, eight rhombomeres can be distinguished from caudal to rostra.

Rh3-Rh1 form the metencephalon and later become the pons cerebellum, a portion of the fourth ventricle and portions of cranial nerves V, VI, VII, VIII.

b) Cranial Fossae

The cranium is divided into three regions (Figure 5.3):

* **Anterior cranial fossa** contains the frontal lobes and includes all of fron-tal and ethmoid bones and the lesser wing of the sphenoid.
* **Middle cranial fossa** contains the temporal lobes and includes the greater wing of the sphenoid, sella turcica and the majority of temporal bones.
* **Posterior cranial fossa** contains the occipital lobes, cerebellum and medulla and includes the occipital bone.

c) Meningeal Layers

Remember *PAD*:

> *P*ia mater = Inner layer
> *A*rachnoid mater = Middle layer
> *D*ura mater = Outer layer

The dura mater is folded to create specific divides between cranial structures:

* **Falx cerebri**: separates the two cerebral hemispheres of the brain.
* **Tentorium cerebelli**: separates the cerebellum from the cerebrum.
* **Falx cerebelli**: separates the cerebellar hemispheres.

DOI: 10.1201/9781003322573-9

Table 5.1 Division of the embryonic brain

Primary brain vesicle	Secondary brain vesicle	Adult brain structures
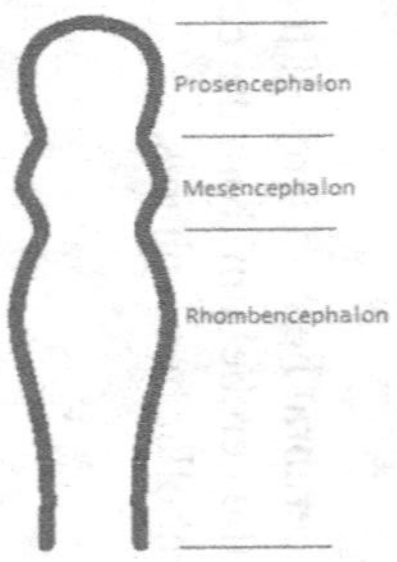 *Prosencephalon* (forebrain) differentiates into:	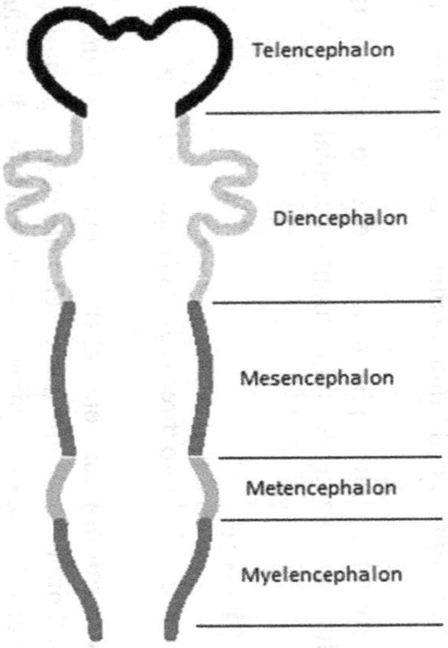 Telencephalon	Cerebral cortex, Subcortical white matter, Basal ganglia, Basal forebrain nuclei
	Diencephalon	Thalamus, Hypothalamus, Epithalamus, Subthalamus, Pretectum
Mesencephalon (midbrain)	Mesencephalon	Tectum (or corpora quadrigemina), Tegmentum, Cerebral peduncles, Ventricular mesocoelia, Several nuclei and fasciculi
Rhombencephalon (hindbrain), which can be subdivided into a number of transversal swellings called *rhombomeres (Rh)*	Metencephalon	*Metencephalon* (Rh3-Rh1) Pons, Cerebellum
	Myelencephalon	*Myelencephalon* Medulla oblongata

Figure 5.2 Secondary brain vesicles

Figure 5.1 Primary brain vesicles

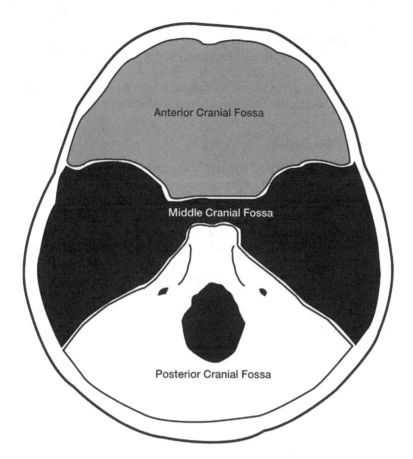

Figure 5.3 Cranial fossae

- **Sellar diaphragm**: covers the pituitary gland and forms a roof over the hypophysial fossa.

d) Cortical Structures

There are four major lobes: frontal, temporal, parietal and occipital.
The lobar surface is folded forming *sulci* (valleys) and *gyri* (ridges).
   Important anatomical landmarks to be aware of include:

- The **central sulcus** (the fissure of Rolando) separates the frontal from the parietal lobe.
- The **lateral sulcus** (the Sylvian fissure) divides the frontal and parietal lobes above from the temporal lobe below.

- The **medial longitudinal fissure** separates the brain into the right and left hemispheres.
- The **precentral gyrus** part of the frontal lobe is the *primary motor cortex*; the representation of different body parts in this region is often termed the homunculus.
- The **postcentral gyrus** part of the parietal lobe is the *primary somatosensory cortex*, with a similar homunculus representation.

Other Major Sulci Include

The **cingulate gyrus** is located on the medial side of the frontal lobe; the anterior portion is considered the *seat of motivation* (Figure 5.4).

The **middle frontal gyrus** constitutes the *dorsolateral prefrontal cortex*, often considered to be responsible for *executive function* (Figure 5.5).

The **inferior parietal lobe** is made of the angular gyrus and the supramarginal gyrus and is considered to be important for *visuospatial* attention (Figure 5.6).

The **superior temporal sulcus** forms the superior temporal gyrus, the seat of the *primary auditory cortex* (Figure 5.7).

The **calcarine sulcus** in the medial occipital cortex is the seat of the *primary visual cortex* (Figure 5.8).

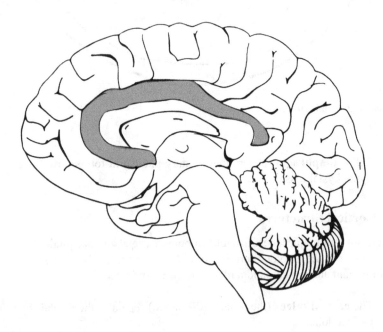

Figure 5.4 Cingulate gyrus

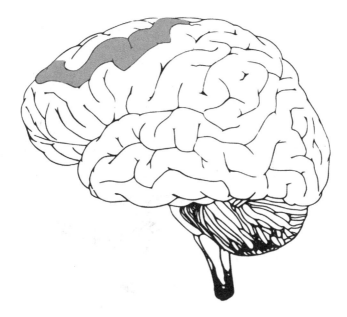

Figure 5.5 Middle frontal gyrus

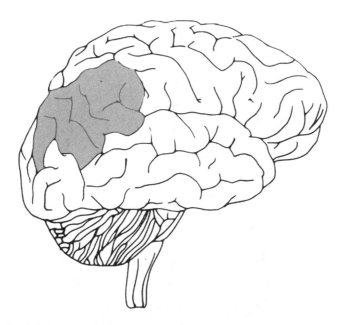

Figure 5.6 Inferior parietal lobe

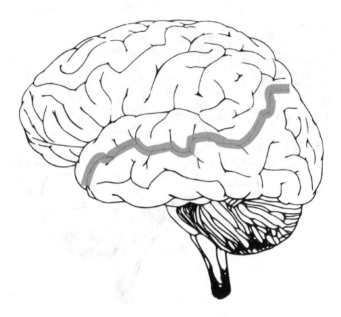

Figure 5.7 Superior temporal sulcus

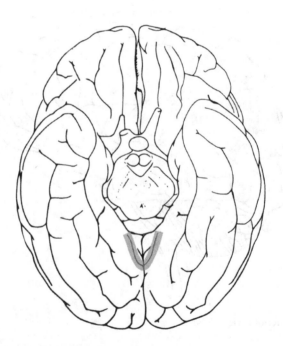

Figure 5.8 The calcarine sulcus

e) Hemispheric Lateralisation

Most fundamental functions of the brain are represented bilaterally; language and comprehension are tending to localise to the left temporal cortex and prosody seems limited to the right (Table 5.2).

The **planum temporale** is located on the surface of the *superior temporal gyrus*. It is *L*arger on the *L*eft than the right hemisphere in *65% of people*. It is probably one of the *most asymmetrical* cranial structures.

It is responsible for *language processing*.

In schizophrenia, this asymmetry is reduced or even reversed.

f) Cranial Foramina

There are multiple foramina in the skull. Table 5.3 includes the most important ones that are likely to crop up in the exams.

g) Subcortical Structures

The **limbic system** is often considered to be evolutionarily older than the higher cortical centres. It has a variety of functions but is primarily responsible for our *behaviour*, *emotion* and *memory*.

The limbic system encompasses many different structures, but the exams tend to focus on a few key elements:

* **Hippocampus**: *memory* processing.
* **Hypothalamus**: influences *neuroendocrine* responses.
* **Nucleus accumbens**: *rewards system* regulation.

Table 5.2 Hemispheric lateralisation of the brain

Left hemisphere lesion	Right hemisphere lesion
Limb apraxia	Constructional apraxia
Dysgraphia (aphasic)	Dysgraphia (spatial, neglect)
Aphasia	Visuospatial defect
Finger agnosia	Neglect
R/L disorientation	Anosognosia
Dyscalculia (number alexia)	Dyscalculia (spatial)
Face Recognition	

Table 5.3 Foramina in the skull

Foramen	Location	Allows passage of
Foramen spinosum	Middle fossa	Middle meningeal artery
Foramen ovale	Middle fossa	Mandibular division of trigeminal nerve
Foramen lacerum	Middle fossa	Internal carotid artery
Foramen magnum	Posterior fossa	Spinal cord
Jugular foramen	Posterior fossa	Cranial nerves IX, X and XI

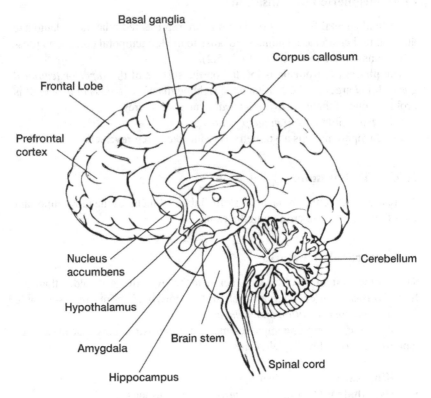

Figure 5.9 Basal ganglia

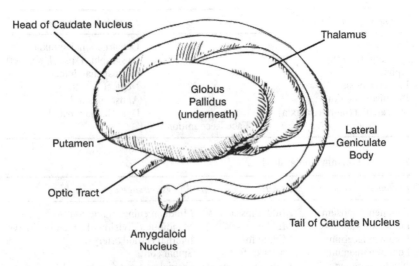

Figure 5.10 Striatum and globus pallidus

The **basal ganglia** are a group of *grey matter* nuclei forming the largest subcortical structure. Their main function is the *planning and programming of movement*, but they may also play a part in some cognitive processes.

The components of the basal ganglia:

* **Striatum** = *caudate nucleus* and *putamen.*
* **Globus pallidus.**

The putamen and globus pallidus are collectively referred to as the *lenticular/lentiform* nucleus.

The **substantia nigra**, divided into *pars compacta*, is located in the mid-brain and has important roles in movement, reward, addiction and mood.

The substantia nigra and the subthalamic nucleus are both functionally related to the basal ganglia but are not considered to be part of it.

Four relevant conditions result from problems with the basal ganglia:

* **Huntington's chorea**: degeneration of the striatum, mainly caudate nucleus.
* **Wilson's disease**: copper deposition in basal ganglia.
* **Parkinson's disease**: degeneration of the substantia nigra.
* **Hemiballism**: decrease in activity of the subthalamic nucleus.

Other conditions relevant to the basal ganglia:

* **Obsessive-compulsive disorder**: higher blood flow and increased metabolism to the caudate nuclei.
* **Tourette's syndrome**: striatal dopaminergic dysfunction.
* **Carbon monoxide poisoning**: bilateral damage to basal ganglia.
* **Fahr's disease**: calcium deposits in the basal ganglia.

h) Thalamus

Think of the thalamus as a large *information processor*, filtering and relaying sensory information from the basal ganglia and cerebellum to the cerebral cortex for processing.

The **hypothalamus** *regulates physiological functions* such as eating, drinking, sleeping and temperature. It contains *chemorecpetors* that monitor glucose levels, osmolarity and acid balance. It pays a key part it in *neuroendocrine* control.

The **ventromedial hypothalamus** acts as the *satiety centre*.

The **lateral hypothalamus** innervates the hypothalamus via *orexinergic neurons,* where its major functions are promoting feeding and arousal.

i) Cerebellum

The cerebellum has the important role of *preparing a motor plan* and *organising muscle groups* so that an action is carried out smoothly.

Functionally it is divided into three regions:

- The anterior and posterior lobes are divided into a medial section, the **spinocerebellum**, allowing for *fine tuned body movements*;
- The lateral section, the **cerebrocerebellum**, involved in planning and *conscious assessment of movement*; and
- The flocculonodular lobe, the **vestibulocerebellum**, responsible for *balance and spatial orientation*.

j) Brain Stem and Cranial Nerves

This is comprised of the *pons*, the *midbrain* and the *medulla*.

Nine out of 12 cranial nerves enter or exit the brain from the brainstem.

The midbrain consists of the **superior** and **inferior colliculi**; the superior is responsible for *conjugate gaze control* and the inferior colliculi for *auditory localisation*.

The substantia nigra is also located in the midbrain.

The pons is positioned beneath the cerebellum and surrounds the upper half of the fourth ventricle.

The medulla surrounds inferior portion of the fourth ventricle.

Cranial Nerve Reflexes

Exam questions might ask which nerves are involved in a specific reflex (Table 5.4).

k) White Matter Pathways

There are three major types of white matter pathways (Table 5.5)

- **Projection fibres**: connect *higher and lower* centres of the brain and run *vertically*.
- **Association fibres**: connect different regions *within the same hemisphere*.
- **Commissural fibres**: connect similar regions *in the opposite hemisphere*.

Table 5.4 Nerves associated with specific reflexes

Reflex	Sensory component	Motor component
Pupillary light reflex	Optic	Oculomotor
Accommodation reflex	Optic	Oculomotor
Jaw jerk	Trigeminal	Trigeminal
Corneal reflex	Trigeminal	Facial
Vestibulo-ocular reflex	Vestibulocochlear	Oculomotor, trochlear, abducens
Gag reflex	Glossopharyngeal	Vagus

Table 5.5 White matter pathways

Tract type	Examples	Description
Projection	Corticospinal	Efferent projection fibres that connect motor cortex to the brain stem and spinal cord
	Corticobulbar	Efferent projection fibres that connect motor cortex to the brain stem and spinal cord
	Corona radiata	Fibres to and from virtually all cortical areas fan out superolaterally from the internal capsule
	Internal capsule	Major conduit of fibres to and from the cerebral cortex
	Geniculocalcarine tract (optic radiation)	Connects the lateral geniculate nucleus to occipital (primary visual) cortex
Commissural	Corpus callosum	The largest bundle, connects the cerebral hemispheres
	Anterior commissure	Interconnects olfactory bulbs
Association	Cingulum	Interconnects portions of the frontal, parietal and temporal lobes
	Superior occipitofrontal fasciculus	Connects occipital and frontal lobes
	Inferior occipitofrontal fasciculus	Connects the occipital and frontal lobes
	Uncinate fasciculus	Connects the orbitofrontal cortex to the anterior and temporal lobes
	Superior longitudinal (arcuate) fasciculus	Connects the frontal lobe cortex to parietal, temporal and occipital lobe cortices (the largest association bundle)
	Inferior longitudinal (occipitotemporal) fasciculus	Connects temporal and occipital lobe cortices

l) Spinal Cord

Unlike the cerebrum that is surrounded by white matter and grey matter on the outer surface, *in the spinal cord, grey matter forms the deepest layer* that surrounds the cerebrospinal fluid, whereas the white matter forms the anterior, lateral and dorsal columns.

* **Dorsal column**: *proprioceptive* sensory fibres.
* **Anterior and lateral columns**: ascending spinothalamic tracts carrying *touch, pressure, pain* and *temperature.*

m) Cerebrospinal Fluid (CSF)

CSF is formed by *ependymal* cells in the *choroid plexus* of the lateral, third and fourth ventricles (approximately 300–500 ml/day).

Route of CSF Passage

CSF passes (Figure 5.11) from the lateral ventricles via the *foramen of Munro* to the third ventricle. From there, it passes via the *aqueduct of Sylvius* (cerebral aqueduct) to the *fourth ventricle*. From the fourth, it passes through the *foramen of Magendie* and *foramen of Luschka* into the *subarachnoid space* and *spinal cord*. It is then reabsorbed by the *arachnoid villi* and enters the dural venous sinuses. Thus, only around 160 ml remains in circuit at any one time.

The normal intra-cerebral pressure (ICP) is *5–15 mm Hg*.

Obstruction of CSF circulation commonly occurs within the third or fourth ventricle, resulting in non-communicating hydrocephalus (*raised ICP*).

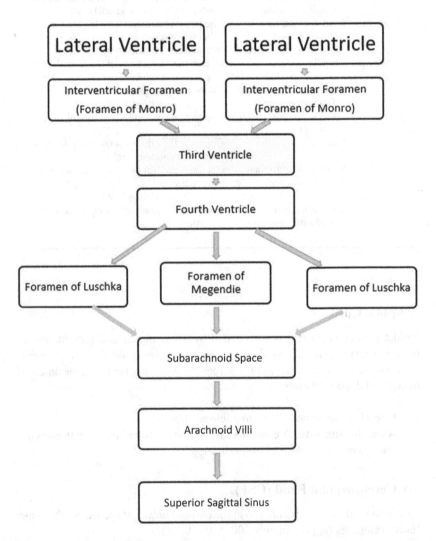

Figure 5.11 Circulation of CSF

Impairment of CSF reabsorption in the subarachnoid space results in communication hydrocephalus (*normal ICP*).

Table 5.6 illustrates the difference in biochemistry between CSF and plasma:

Table 5.6 CSF concentrations relative to the plasma

Reduced	Unchanged	Increased
Protein content	Sodium	Chloride
Glucose		Magnesium
Cholesterol		
pH		
Calcium		
Potassium		

There are no lymphatic channels in the brain, and CSF fulfils the role of returning interstitial fluid and protein to the circulation.

The CSF is separated from blood by the blood-brain barrier. Only *lipid soluble substances* can easily cross, which is essential to maintaining the integrity of the border between blood and brain.

n) Blood Supply

The body supplies blood to the brain via the *internal carotid* and *vertebral arteries*. These vessels come together to form a ring called the *circle of Willis*, a network which provides a *collateral system* should any of the vessels become damaged.

Arising from the circle are the three main vessels that supply the brain with blood:

- **Anterior cerebral artery**
- **Middle cerebral artery**
- **Posterior cerebral artery**

Exam questions will test your anatomy knowledge but also want you to have an understanding of the functional damage that might result in an occlusion of each of the arteries.

The **anterior cerebral artery** (ACA) supplies the *medial* and *superior* tip of the *lateral aspect* of the cerebral cortex up to the *parietal/occipital border*.

Occlusion of the ACA may result in the following defects:

- Hemiparesis of the contralateral foot and leg more than the arm
- Sensory loss of the contralateral foot and leg
- Motor dysphasia

The **middle cerebral artery** (MCA) supplies most of the *lateral* aspects of the *cerebral cortex* up to the *border of the occipital and parietal lobe*.

Occlusion of the MCA may result in the following defects:

- Hemiparesis of the contralateral face and limbs
- Sensory loss of contralateral face and limbs
- Dysphasia (when dominant hemisphere affected)
- Contralateral neglect
- Homonymous hemianopia or quadrantanopia
- Dorsolateral prefrontal dysfunction

The **posterior cerebral artery** (PCA) arises from the **basilar artery** and supplies the *inferomedial temporal lobe* and the *occipital lobe*.

Occlusion of the PCA may result in the following defects:

- Alexia without agraphia (left PCA)
- Contralateral loss of pain and temperature sensation
- Contralateral hemianopia
- Prosopagnosia
- Ipsilateral cranial nerve defects (V, VIII, IX, X, XI)
- Horner's syndrome

The *medulla* is supplied by the **posterior inferior cerebellar arteries** (PICA) and the **anterior spinal branches** of the vertebral arteries.

Pons is supplied by the **basilar artery** that runs along the midline of the pons.

o) Blood-Brain Barrier (BBB)

The BBB acts as the brain's security system, allowing passage of essential nutrients but blocking harmful chemicals. It is formed by the formation of *tight junctions* between endothelial cells in the capillaries of the brain, separating the brain from the CSF.

At several parts of the brain, the BBB is *fenestrated* to allow permeation of neurosecretory products to enter the blood. These areas are known as the *circumventricular organs*:

- Posterior pituitary
- Pineal body

- Area postrema
- Subfornical organ
- Median eminence
- Vascular organ of the lamina terminalis

Exam questions will normally focus on the following points:

- *Lipid soluble* molecules are able to pass through much more easily than water soluble molecules.
- The BBB is less effective and more permeable when inflamed.
- Molecules that are *highly charged* and *very large* will struggle to pass through.
- *Nasal preparations* can theoretically bypass the BBB.

Source Material

Kumar, Parveen, and Michael L. Clark. (2016). *Kumar and Clark's Clinical Medicine*. London: Elsevier, 9th ed., pp. 0–1456.

Martin, John H. (18 July 2012). *Neuroanatomy Text and Atlas*. New York: McGraw-Hill Education – Europe, 4th ed., pp. 0–528.

Martini, Frederic H., Judi L. Nath, and Edwin F. Bartholomew. (2017). *Fundamentals of Anatomy & Physiology*. London: Pearson, 11th ed., pp. 0–1296.

Tortora, Gerard J., and Bryan H. Derrickson. (2014). *Principles of Anatomy and Physiology*. London: John Wiley & Sons.

Willis, T. (1963). In W. Feindel (Ed.), *The Anatomy of the Brain and Nerves*. Montreal: McGill University Press.

6 Neurophysiology

Elizabeth Templeton

a) The Action Potential
b) The Hypothalamic-Pituitary-Adrenal Axis (HPA)
c) Adrenal Fatigue
d) Thyroid Gland
e) Adrenal Cortex
f) Dexamethasone Suppression Tests (DSTs)
g) Tremors
h) Electroencephalograms (EEG)
i) Sleep Architecture
j) Sleep Disorders

a) The Action Potential

Generation of an **action potential** along a neuron takes place in five steps:

- A stimulus from a sensory cell or another neuron causes the *membrane* to *depolarise* (become more positive) towards the threshold potential.
- Once the threshold is reached, the *sodium ion* (Na+) *channels open* to allow sodium ions to rush into the cell.
- At the peak of the action potential, the *potassium channels* start to *open* at the same time the *sodium channels* start to *close*.
- The cell become *hyperpolarised* (becomes more negative) as the *potassium ions (K+) leave* the cell. During this phase, the cell becomes *refractory* and is unable to fire again (depolarise).
- The *potassium channels close* and the cell is restored to its *resting membrane potential* with the help of the *Na+/K+ transporter*.

b) The Hypothalamic-Pituitary-Adrenal Axis (HPA)

The HPA can be thought of as the *stress response system*.

Neuroendocrine production occurs at the sites set out in Table 6.1.

The HPA also helps to *regulate bodily systems* such as digestion, immunity, sexuality, energy and emotions.

DOI: 10.1201/9781003322573-10

Table 6.1 Sites of neuroendocrine production

Anterior pituitary	• Growth hormone (GH)
	• Thyroid stimulating hormone (TSH)
	• Follicle stimulating hormone (FSH)
	• Adreno corticotrophin hormone (ACTH)
	• Luteinising hormone (LH)
Posterior pituitary	• Oxytocin
	• Vasopressin
Hypothalamus	• Corticotrophin releasing hormone (CRH)
	• Thyrotrophin releasing hormone (TRH)
	• Prolactin inhibitory factor (PIF)
	• Somatostatin (SST)
	• Growth hormone releasing hormone (GHRH)
	• Gonadotrophin releasing hormone (GnRH)
Adrenal gland	• Cortisol
	• Adrenaline
	• Noradrenaline
	• Aldosterone

When feeling stressed, either thinking about an exam or being confronted by a wild animal:

- The hypothalamus releases CRH, which targets the pituitary gland.
- The pituitary in turn releases ACTH, which acts on the adrenal glands.
- The adrenals then release cortisol.
- The role of cortisol is to mobilise the body's energy reserves (fight mode) by raising sugar levels in the blood. The adrenal gland assists by increasing heart rate and blood pressure.
- These hormones work on a negative feedback loop so the hypothalamus can detect the rise in cortisol, which inhibits further release of CRH.

c) Adrenal Fatigue

In subjects who are chronically stressed (observed in patients suffering with post-traumatic stress disorder [PTSD]) such that a state of 'adrenal exhaustion' can be reached where the adrenal glands become so depleted of cortisol, that there is inadequate release in response to stress. This can be identified clinically by an overall drop in blood serum levels.

Low cortisol levels are also seen in chronic fatigue and fibromyalgia.

Hypercortisolaemia has been seen in some patients with mania, OCD and disorders like schizoaffective disorders.

d) Thyroid Gland

- The hypothalamus releases TRH, which stimulates TSH from the pituitary.

Table 6.2 Features of thyroid gland dysfunction

Hypothyroidism	• Fatigue
	• Weight gain
	• Cold intolerance
	• Dry skin
	• Psychomotor retardation
	• Reduced libido
	• Poor memory
	• It has been implicated in rapid cycling disorders
Hyperthyroidism	• Tachycardia
	• Weight loss
	• Heat intolerance
	• Sweating
	• Anxiety
	• Irritability
	• Poor concentration
	• Agitation
	• Emotional lability

- TSH stimulates the thyroid gland to produce thyroxine (T4) and triiodothyro-nine (T3). *T3 is more potent*, with T4 being converted into T3 by target organs.

In depression, a blunted response to TRH release is observed, with some evidence to suggest that adding T3 and T4 supplements to antidepressant treatment could improve responsiveness.

Features of thyroid gland dysfunction is outlined in Table 6.2.

e) Adrenal Cortex

- The hypothalamus releases CRH, which stimulates the anterior pituitary to release ACTH.
- ACTH stimulates the adrenal cortex to release cortisol.
- This in turn inhibits the release of both CRH and ACTH.

Features of adrenal gland dysfunction are outlined in Table 6.3.

Post-Traumatic Stress Disorder

In patients with PTSD, ambient cortisol levels are lower than normal. This state has been attributed to chronic inhibition of the HPA axis by persistent severe anxiety.

f) Dexamethasone Suppression Tests (DSTs)

Exogenous corticosteroids like dexamethasone will suppress endogenous cortisol production if the HPA is intact. If not, a cortisol level greater than 5 mcg/L will be measured following administration of DST.

Non-suppression is seen in *depression* and *Cushing's syndrome*.

Table 6.3 Features of adrenal gland dysfunction

Cushing's disease (low cortisol)	• Fatigue • Weight loss • Cold intolerance • Dry skin • Confusion • Depression • Mania • Psychosis
Addison's disease (raised cortisol)	• Hyperpigmentation • Apathy • Fatigue • Depression • Irritability • Anxiety • Emotional lability

g) Tremors

Types of tremor are outlined in Table 6.4.

Table 6.4 Types of tremor

Psychogenic tremor	Changeable nature; often *responds to distraction*.
Parkinsonian tremor	Classically described as *pill rolling*, occurs *at rest* at a frequency of *5 Hz*. Associated with Parkinson's disease.
Benign essential tremor	Can be related to heightened emotions with no underlying pathology. Typically begins in the fourth decade of life. It can involve the hands, legs, body and head. The frequency is *7 Hz*.
Cerebellar tremor	An intention tremor; worsens with *purposeful movement*.
Physiological tremor	Induced when trying to hold a specific posture. It is very fine and may not be visible to the naked eye. It can be pronounced in states of heightened arousal. The frequency is *10 Hz*.

h) Electroencephalograms (EEG)

EEG wave patterns are outlined in Table 6.5.
 Beta and alpha are considered fast waves.
 Theta and delta are considered slow waves.
 Certain conditions are associated with specific EEG changes, as in Table 6.6.
 Drugs can be associated with EEG effects, as in Table 6.7 and Table 6.8.

i) Sleep Architecture

 NREM = non-rapid eye movement; *synchronised* sleep.
 REM = rapid eye movement; *desynchronised* sleep.

Table 6.5 EEG wave patterns

Type	Frequency	Notes
Delta	1–4 Hz	Associated with *sleep*, pathological in an awake state, common in deeper sleep.
Theta	4–8 Hz	Associated with *light sleep* in children and drowsy adults, pathological in an awake state, *fronto-temporal area.*
Alpha	8–12 Hz	Associated with an *awake but relaxed* state when eyes are closed, reduced with anxiety, eye opening or concentration, reduced with age, *occipito-parietal area.*
Beta	12–30 Hz	Associated with an *awake* state, *frontal position.*
Gamma	30–100 Hz	Associated with *meditation.*

Table 6.6 Conditions associated with specific EEG changes

Condition	EEG findings
Creutzfeldt–Jakob disease (CJD) (sporadic only, does not apply to acquired variant CJD)	Periodic biphasic (1–2 Hz) and triphasic synchronous sharp wave complexes superimposed on a slow background rhythm.
Huntington's disease	Initial loss of alpha and later flattened trace.
Delirium	Diffuse slowing, increased delta and theta, reduced alpha.
Delirium tremens	Hyperactive trace, fast.
Alzheimer's disease	Rarely normal in advanced dementia, reduced alpha and beta, increased delta and theta. Could be useful to differentiate pseudodementia.
Petit mal epilepsy (absence seizure)	3 Hz (3 waves per second) spike and wave pattern.
Generalised epilepsy	Sharp spikes, 25–30 Hz.
Partial epilepsy	Focal spikes.
Myoclonic epilepsy	Spike and wave activity.
Encephalopathy	Diffuse slowing.
Normal aging	Focal (temporal region) or diffuse slowing.
Angelman syndrome	EEG changes notable by age 2, occipital 4–6 Hz activity with eye closure seen under the age of 12, runs of 1–2 Hz high amplitude frontal activity with superimposed interictal epileptiform discharges seen in all ages.
Encephalopathy	Diffuse slowing.
Mass lesion	Focal slowing.

Table 6.7 EEG effects associated with recreational drugs

Recreational drugs	EEG changes
Stimulants amphetamine, cocaine, nicotine	Increase alpha.
Caffeine	In withdrawal, increase theta.
Cannabis	Incrase alpha.
Depressants alcohol, opioids	Decrease alpha.

Table 6.8 EEG effects associated with psychotropic drugs

Psychotropics	EEG changes
Antipsychotics typical Haloperidol least effect	Decreased beta with increased alpha, theta and delta.
Antipsychotics atypical Clozapine significant effect	Varied.
Antidepressants	Reduced beta, increased alpha, theta and delta.
Anticonvulsants	Nil effect.
Lithium	Generalised slowing.
Benzodiazepines	Decreased alpha, increased beta.
Opioids	Decreased alpha, increased theta and delta, slow waves are seen in OD.
Barbiturates	Increased beta.

Features of NREM sleep:

- 75% of sleep is NREM
- Reduced physiological functions:
    - Decreased heart rate
    - Decreased systolic blood pressure
    - Decreased respiratory rate
    - Decreased cerebral blood flow
    - Reduced recall of dreams if woken (sleep terror is a NREM sleep disorder seen in children, once woken they cannot remember the event, *unlike a nightmare*)
    - Abolition of tendon reflexes
    - Upward ocular deviation with few or no eye movements
    - Penis not usually erect

NREM consists of four stages (Table 6.9). Time from stage 1–4 is normally 20 minutes. Stages 3–4 constitute slow wave sleep (SWS).

REM Sleep

- Twenty-five percent of adult sleep is REM sleep.

Table 6.9 Stages of NREM sleep

Stage 1	Drowsy period—transition between wakefulness and sleep.
	Decreased reactivity to external stimuli, but if woken from this stage of sleep, individual will deny being asleep.
	EEG shows *low voltage theta* activity: 3–17 Hz.
	5% of sleep.
Stage 2	Thought processes become further fragmented.
	EEG shows *sleep spindles* and *K complexes*.
	45% of sleep.
Stage 3	Nocturnal enuresis more likely to occur.
	Slow wave/deep sleep.
	EEG shows *delta waves*.
Stage 4	Physiological functions are at their lowest.
	EEG shows *delta waves >50%* of the time.

- *Darting eye movements* are noted in REM sleep despite other *muscles being paralysed*.
- Occurs in 90-minute intervals and is associated with a high level of brain activity.
- In REM sleep disorder, muscle paralysis is impaired, which can lead to violent incidents with patients enacting out their dreams.
- EEG patterns show:

    - Mixed frequency low voltage waves
    - Saw tooth pattern

Features of REM Sleep

- Increased sympathetic functions
- Increased heart rate (HR)
- Increased blood pressure (BP)
- Increased respiratory rate (RR)
- Increased cerebral blood flow
- Increased protein synthesis
- Loss of muscle tone
- Vivid recall of dreams

Brain Activity

Apart from oscillatory background patterns, there are some specific sleep patterns to be aware of:

K complexes: large amplitude delta frequency waves, sometimes with a sharp apex that occurs when a person is *aroused from sleep*.

Sleep spindles: the waveform resembles a spindle, seen predominantly in *stage 2* sleep.

V waves: occur during sleep particularly at *stage 2*, usually symmetrical.

j) Sleep Disorders

Dyssomnias are *primary* disorders of falling asleep or staying asleep, or of excessive sleepiness, and are characterised by a disturbance in the quality, timing or amount of sleep.

They can be intrinsic, meaning organic, or extrinsic, related to the person's environment, as in Table 6.10.

Intrinsic Sleep Disorders

Narcolepsy

- Aetiology is unknown.
- Onset is in the second decade, with a peak at the age of 14 years.
- Chronic brain disorder that involves poor control of sleep wake cycles.
- Characterised by *excessive daytime sleepiness*, with sudden bouts of irresistible sleep that can strike at any time and typically last a few seconds to several minutes.
- The sleep attacks can occur in situations never normally associated with falling asleep, such as interviews/exams.
- Normally *associated with cataplexy*, sudden loss of bilateral muscle tone provoked by strong emotion.
- Once the subject wakes, they feel refreshed but quickly start to feel sleepy again and the cycles repeats.
- Sufferers often experience nocturnal disruption, hypnogogic hallucinations and sleep paralysis.
- Investigations for diagnosis include *sleep deprived EEG*, *polysomnogram*, *multiple sleep latency* and *CSF* in selected cases.

Table 6.10 Dyssomnias and parasomnias

Main class	Subcategory	Important examples
Dyssomnias	Extrinsic sleep disorders	Inadequate sleep hygiene, alcohol dependent sleep disorder
	Intrinsic sleep disorders	Narcolepsy, idiopathic hypersomnia, restless leg syndrome, periodic limb movement disorder, obstructive sleep apnoea
	Circadian rhythm disorders	Jet lag syndrome, shift work sleep disorder, irregular sleep/wake pattern, delayed sleep phase syndrome, advanced sleep phase disorder
Parasomnias	Arousal disorders	Sleep walking, sleep terrors
	Sleep wake transition disorders	Rhythmic movement disorder, sleep talking, nocturnal leg cramps
	Parasomnias associated with REM sleep	Nightmares, sleep paralysis
	Other parasomnias	Sleep bruxism

- Treatment with regular dose *amphetamine* and *methylphenidate*. Tricyclics are used to treat cataplexy.

Periodic Limb Movement Disorder

- Repetitive cramping or jerking of the legs during sleep.
- Movements are repetitive and rhythmic, occurring about very 20–40 seconds.
- The movements can be associated with awakening or partial arousal. If the subject is aware of the sleep disruption, they might complain of excessive day time sleepiness.

Restless Leg Syndrome (RLS)

- RLS is a neurological disorder characterised by an irresistible urge to move your legs.
- Genetics thought to be important; 50% of subjects have a relative with RLS.
- The sensation is completely relieved on completion of leg motion but returns again soon after.
- The sensation is normally worse when lying down.
- For many people, it causes sleep disruption.
- Risk factors include women, middle/older age, pregnancy, renal failure, iron deficiency anaemia, vitamin B12 deficiency, peripheral neuropathy, certain antipsychotic and antidepressant medications.

Rhythmic Movement Disorder

- Characterised by large stereotyped repetitive movements involving large muscles usually of the head or neck.
- Repeated head banging is a common presentation.
- Most subjects are otherwise healthy infants or children; however, it can be associated with autism or mental retardation and other pathology if it persists into adulthood.

Arousal Disorders

SLEEP TERRORS

- Characterised by sudden arousal from sleep with a sense of terror or dread.
- Associated with an autonomic fear response: tachycardia, flushing, sweating, tachypnoea.
- Usually occurs during *stage 3–4 NREM sleep*.
- Subject remains asleep and can become disorientated if awoken.
- Subjects typically cannot recall episode the following morning.

Note: nightmares often occur later in the night. They may wake the subject, who can often recall some of the context and be able to describe it.

SLEEP WALKING (SOMNAMBULISM)

- An automatism occurring in slow wave sleep, so within NREM sleep.
- Sleep walking can start in childhood and is most common between the ages of 5–12 years.
- Associated with enuresis.
- The behaviours might range from simply sitting up in bed to roaming beyond the room.
- Typically, subjects are hard to wake and will be confused and disorientated when awoken.
- There is likely a genetic component.

SLEEP PARALYSIS

- Transient paralysis of skeletal muscles, rendering the subject unable to move or speak.
- Typically occurs when a person is falling asleep or waking up from sleep.
- Can be associated with hallucinations.
- Genetics and sleep deprivation thought to be risk factors for sleep paralysis. It has also been linked with narcolepsy, migraines, anxiety disorders and obstructive sleep apnoea.
- If severe, clonazepam can be used.

Source Material

Goroll, Allan H., and Albert G. Mulley. (1 January 2009). *Primary Care Medicine: Office Evaluation and Management of the Adult Patient.* Philadelphia: Lippincott Williams & Wilkins, p. 1178.

Hirshkowitz, Max. (2004). *Chapter 10, Neuropsychiatric Aspects of Sleep and Sleep Disorders.* Arlington, VA: American Psychiatric Publishing, pp. 315–340.

Kumar, Parveen, and Michael L. Clark. (2016). *Kumar and Clark's Clinical Medicine.* London: Elsevier, 9th ed., pp. 0–1456.

Martin, John H. (18 July 2012). *Neuroanatomy Text and Atlas.* New York: McGraw-Hill Education – Europe, 4th ed., pp. 0–528.

Martini, Frederic H., Judi L. Nath, and Edwin F. Bartholomew. (2017). *Fundamentals of Anatomy & Physiology.* London: Pearson, 11th ed., pp. 0–1296.

Niedermeyer, E., and da Silva, F. L. (2004). *Electroencephalography: Basic Principles, Clinical Applications, and Related Fields.* Philadelphia: Lippincott Williams & Wilkins.

Panayiotopoulos, C. P. (2010). *A Clinical Guide to Epileptic Syndromes and Their Treatment.* London: Springer-Verlag, 2nd ed., pp. 0–578.

Tatum, William O. (2014). *Handbook of EEG Interpretation.* New York: Demos Medical Publishing, pp. 155–190.

Tortora, Gerard J., and Bryan H. Derrickson. (2014). *Principles of Anatomy and Physiology.* London: John Wiley & Sons, pp. 0–1300.

7 Neurochemistry

Elizabeth Templeton

a) Classification of Receptors

- **Ionotropic ligand gated channels** result in a *fast* response by opening ion channels on the cell surface. The effects are generally short lived.
- **G coupled metabotropic receptors** are relatively *slower*.

Table 7.1 outlines the classes of some common receptors.

Neurotransmitters can be classified into excitatory and inhibitory forms, as in Table 7.2.

b) Biogenic Amines

Serotonin plays an important role in many functions, including control of anger, mood, sleep, aggression, sexuality and appetite.

Tryptophan is the precursor to serotonin.

It is *converted to 5-HTP* (5 hydroxytryptophan) via the enzyme *tryptophan hydroxylase*.

5-HTP is further *decarboxylated* to *serotonin* by *aromatic L-amino acid decarboxylase*.

Many illicit substances block the reuptake of serotonin to the synapse: methylenedioxymethamphetamine (MDMA), amphetamine, cocaine and of course medications such as selective serotonin reuptake inhibitors (SSRIs) and tricyclic antidepressants (TCAs).

Serotonin is metabolised by monoamine oxidase (MAO) enzymes and aldehyde dehydrogenase to form 5-HIAA (5-hydroxyindoleacetic acid), which can be excreted via the kidneys.

It has been observed that subjects with low levels of 5 HIAA in their CSF are more likely to commit suicide and respond less well to antidepressant therapy.

Receptors

There are 14 different types of serotonin receptors:

- All are *G-coupled* except 5-HT3, which is ligand gated.

DOI: 10.1201/9781003322573-11

Table 7.1 Common receptor classes

Ionotopic	Metabotropic
Glycine	Adrenergic
Glutaminergic	Dopaminergic
N-methyl-D-aspartate	
(NMDA)	
5HT—3	Serotonergic (except 5HT3)
GABA A	GABA B
Nicotinic	Muscarinic

Table 7.2 Excitatory and inhibitory neurotransmitters

Acetylcholine	Excitatory
Adrenaline	Excitatory
Noradrenaline	Excitatory
Serotonin	Excitatory
Glutamate	Excitatory
Dopamine	Excitatory and inhibitory
Glycine	Mainly inhibitory
Gamma-aminobutyric acid (GABA)	Inhibitory

- Activation of 5-HT2 receptors can have an *antipsychotic* effect and cause sedation.
- 5-HT3 can be associated with *nausea* (antagonism can produce an antiemetic effect).
- 5-HT7 is responsible for the *circadian rhythm*.

Histamine

- Histidine amino acid is converted to histamine via histidine decarboxylase.
- Histamine is metabolised by MAO and methyltransferase.

Histamine exerts its actions by combining with the histamine receptors in Table 7.3.

c) Catecholamines

Dopamine

First synthesised in vitro by George **Barger** and James **Evans** in 1910, its role as a neurotransmitter was discovered by Arvid **Carlsson**, who won the Nobel Prize for it in 1958.

Dopamine is derived from *tyrosine*.

Tyrosine is converted to L-Dopa by the enzyme tyrosine hydroxylase.

L-Dopa is converted to dopamine by the enzyme dopa-decarboxylase.

Table 7.3 Histamine receptors

Histamine receptor	Location	Function
H1	Central nervous system (CNS) tissue, smooth muscle and endothelium	Vasodilation, bronchoconstriction, pain and itching from stings
H2	Parietal cells in stomach	Stimulates gastric acid secretion
H3	Central and peripheral nervous tissue	Decreases the release of other neurotransmitters (serotonin, noradrenaline, acetylcholine)
H4	Basophils	Chemotaxis (cellular movement)

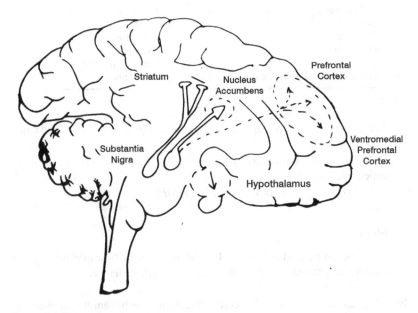

Figure 7.1 Dopaminergic systems

Dopamine is broken down by *catechol-O-methyl transferase* (*COMT*) and MAO; MAO-B more commonly, as MAO-A is more selective towards serotonin and noradrenaline.

Dopamine is *stored in synaptic vesicles* within dopaminergic neurons that travel down the axon toward the terminal until it is released by an action potential.

Dopaminergic neurons are found in four main systems within the brain (Figure 7.1).

The **nigrostriatal system** plays an important role in the control of *movement*. Neurons of the nigrostriatal system originate in the *substantia nigra* and terminate in the *caudate nucleus* and *putamen.*

Blockages of dopamine receptors in this pathway are thought to produce *extrapyramidal side effects (EPSEs).*

The **mesolimbic system** plays an important role in reinforcing (*rewarding*) the effects of using drugs. The mesolimbic system originates in the *ventral tegmental area (VTA)* and projects to several parts of the *limbic system, nucleus accumbens, amygdala* and *hippocampus.*

Blockage of D2 receptors in this pathway is thought to account for the *therapeutic* benefits of antipsychotic medication.

The **mesocortical system** is involved in *planning* and *problem solving.* It originates in the *VTA* and projects dopaminergic axons to the *prefrontal cortex.*

Decreased activity in this pathway is thought to lead to the *negative,* cognitive and affective symptoms of schizophrenia.

The **tuberoinfundibular pathway** is necessary to stimulate prolactin release. It originates in the *arcuate nucleus* of the hypothalamus, projecting into the anterior pituitary.

Blockade of dopamine receptors in this pathway will lead to *hyperprolactinaemia* and therefore lactation, disturbed menstrual cycles, sexual dysfunction and, in the long term, osteoporosis.

There are five types of **dopamine receptors**—D1, D2, D3, D4 and D5—divided into two categories:

* D1-like = D1+D5

  * *Activates* adenylate cyclase (*excitatory*).
* D2-like = D2+D3+D4
  * *Decreases* adenylate cyclase (*inhibitory*).

All types of dopamine receptors are *G coupled.*

Noradrenaline (NA)

Noradrenaline plays a central role in controlling *memory, attention*, rest cycles and *alertness* in the CNS.

Noradrenergic neurons can be found mostly in the *pons, medulla* and *thalamus.*

The main site of NA release is from the *locus coeruleus* in the pons.

NA is derived from *tyrosine* and is synthesised after dopamine.

Once dopamine has been stored in synaptic vesicles, it is converted into NA by dopamine B-hydroxylase.

NA is then converted into adrenaline by phenylethanolamine-N-methyltransferase.

Metabolism is via MAO-A and catechol-O-methyltransferase (COMT).

NA is involved with two major types:

- α1 and α2—α1 is *C-coupled* and mainly *post synaptic*; α2 is *G-coupled* and mostly *presynaptic*.
- β1 and β2—both are *G-coupled*. They have a higher affinity to NA than adrenaline and are found at the *locus coeruleus*.

d) Monoamine Oxidase (MAO)

MAO occurs in two forms:

- **MAO-A** metabolises dopamine, serotonin, noradrenaline, adrenaline and melatonin.
- **MAO-B** metabolises dopamine and phenethylamine.

e) Acetylcholine

Acetylcholine was the first neurotransmitter to be discovered. It acts both centrally and peripherally.

It is synthesised via the enzyme choline acetyltransferase, which transfers an acetyl group from acetyl co-enzyme-A to choline, forming acetylcholine.

Acetylcholine is metabolised by acetylcholinesterase.

There are two main receptor types:

- **Nicotinic**: *ionotropic* receptors stimulated by nicotine and acetylcholine
- **Muscarinic**: *G-coupled* receptors

    There are five different types, M1—M5, which are stimulated by muscarine and acetylcholine.

Source Material

Kumar, Parveen, and Michael L. Clark. (2016). *Kumar and Clark's Clinical Medicine*. London: Elsevier, 9th ed., pp. 0–1456.

Martin, John H. (18 July 2012). *Neuroanatomy Text and Atlas*. New York: McGraw-Hill Education – Europe, 4th ed., pp. 0–528.

Tortora, Gerard J., and Bryan H. Derrickson. (2014). *Principles of Anatomy and Physiology*. London: John Wiley & Sons. 0–1300.

Willis, T. (1963). In W. Feindel (Ed.), *The Anatomy of the Brain and Nerves*. Montreal: McGill University Press.

8 Molecular Genetics

Elizabeth Templeton

a) DNA

DNA is *double stranded* and is composed of many nucleotides. Each nucleotide consists of:

- A *phosphate* group
- A *deoxyribose* sugar
- A *nitrogenous* base (adenine *A*, guanine *G*, pyrimidine (thymine) *T* and cytosine *C*)

Each nucleotide is a base joined to a sugar phosphate unit. The two strands of DNA are held together by hydrogen bonds that form between the nitrogenous bases.

There are only four ways in which the bases will pair: TA, AT, GC, CG.

Gene: this is a portion of DNA that codes for a specific polypeptide sequence. The length of each gene depends on the size of the polypeptide coded.

Codon: a set of three adjacent nucleotides (*triplets*), each coding for an amino acid. Humans have 20 amino acids, ten of which are said to be 'essential', as they are not found in our diet and need to be synthesised. However, there are 64 possible codon combinations, meaning that different triplets might code for the same amino acid. Codons are used as signals in the genetic code, where they might terminate or initiate a polypeptide chain synthesis.

Exon: polypeptide coding sequence in DNA.

Intron: non-coding *junk* sequence, removed from the messenger RNA before it leaves the nucleus and starts protein synthesis. The introns contain three types of sequences, termed satellite, minisatellite and microsatellite.

b) RNA

RNA is *single stranded* and is made up of the same components as DNA, but there are some important differences to be aware of:

- RNA nucleotides *contain ribose*, whilst DNA contains deoxyribose.

DOI: 10.1201/9781003322573-12

- RNA has the base *uracil* rather than the thymine that is present in DNA.
- RNA is usually much *shorter* than DNA.

c) Copying DNA

Replication: refers to the production of new DNA copies from template copies of DNA.

Transcription: refers to the *synthesis of RNA* from nuclear DNA, which occurs within the cell's nucleus.

RNA synthesised during transcription contains introns, which do not code for polypeptides. This unprepared RNA undergoes *splicing* to remove the introns and becomes messenger RNA (mRNA).

Transfer RNA is also synthesised from DNA but in a separate process.

The mRNA then leaves the cell nucleus and enters the cytoplasm, where it directs the synthesis of proteins.

Translation: refers to the process of translating the mRNA sequences into amino acids and then polypeptide chains. In the cell cytoplasm, *ribosomes* read the sequence of the mRNA in groups of three bases to assemble a protein. Termination of this chain occurs when the ribosomes read a 'stop codon' signalled by the combination of either UAA, UGA or UAG.

Figure 8.1 provides a diagram of the process of transcription and translation.

d) DNA Mutations

A mutation is a *heritable change* in the DNA sequence that will ultimately be copied into the mRNA sequence and translated into proteins leading to disease.

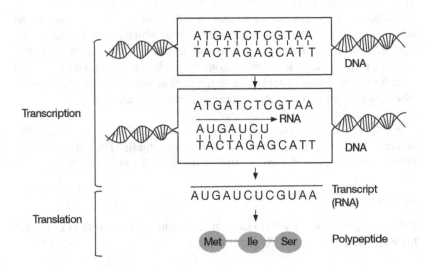

Figure 8.1 DNA transcription and translation

Point mutation refers to a *single base alteration*. Point mutations can manifest in three different ways:

• **Silent mutation**: where the altered codon codes for the same amino acid (no affect).
• **Missense mutation**: where the altered codon codes for a different amino acid.
• **Nonsense**: where the altered codon codes for a stop signal.

According to the effect on the triplet sequence, mutations can be described as 'frame shift' or 'in frame' mutations:

Frame shift mutation: the deletion or insertion is not in multiples of three codons, for example, a segment of five bases is deleted, which creates a shift in the way triplets are read and can have significant effects.

In frame mutation: the deletion or insertion happens in multiples of three codons, with no disturbance in the actual reading frame.

e) Translocations

Translocation refers to the exchange of genetic material in which a chromosome breaks and a portion of it reattaches to a different chromosome. They are mostly *reciprocal*, so one segment is swapped for another.

Robertsonian translocations (Figure 8.2) are *non-reciprocal*, so there is an unequal exchange of genetic material. This results in a single fused

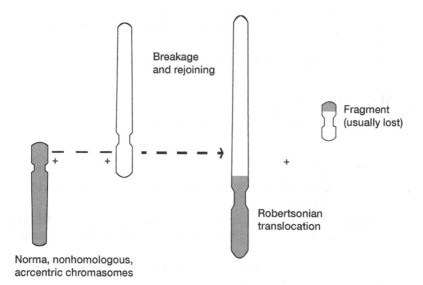

Figure 8.2 Robertsonian translocation

chromosome. Chromosomes in Robertsonian translocations typically involve *acrocentric chromosomes* (very small p-arms). The two p-arms are discarded, and a *metacentric* chromosome is produced with only a small loss of genetic material.

Robertsonian translocations are considered to be balanced and viable.

However, when a gamete is formed, only one gamete will receive the new metacentric chromosome, resulting in monosomy (unbalanced transloca-tion). This is one of the mechanisms of *Down syndrome*. If the mother is a carrier of such translocation, the recurrence rate of Down syndrome is extremely high.

f) Terminology

Allele: one of two or more forms a gene may take.

Dominant: an allele whose expression overpowers the effect of a second form of the same gene.

Gamete: a reproductive cell.

Heterozygous: a condition in which two alleles for a given gene are differ-ent from each other (Dd, Dd).

Homozygous: a condition in which two alleles for a given gene are the same (dd, DD).

Recessive: an allele whose effects are concealed in offspring by the domi-nant allele in the pair.

Phenotype: an individual's observable traits, such as height, eye colour and blood type. The phenotype results from the interaction between the genotype and the environment.

Genotype: an individual's collection of genes.

Haplotype: a set of DNA variations, or polymorphisms, that tend to be inherited together.

Karyotype: an individual's collection of chromosomes.

g) Mendelian Inheritance

There are four types of Mendelian inheritance patterns.

Autosomal Dominant (AD)

Dominant conditions are expressed in individuals who have just one copy of the mutant allele (Figure 8.2).

Affected individuals have one normal copy of the gene and one mutant copy of the gene; thus, each offspring has a 50% chance of inheriting the mutant copy.

Examples of AD conditions include Marfan syndrome, Huntington's dis-ease, achondroplasia and neurofibromatosis.

Autosomal dominant

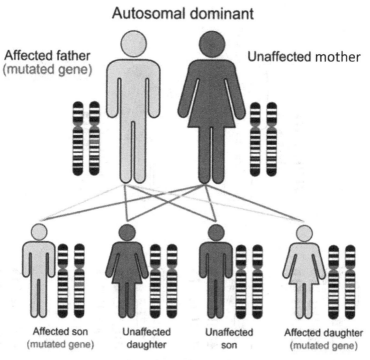

Affected father
(mutated gene)

Unaffected mother

Affected son
(mutated gene)

Unaffected
daughter

Unaffected
son

Affected daughter
(mutated gene)

Probabilities: 1:2

Figure 8.3 Autosomal dominant

Source: Kuebi = Armin Kübelbeck, CC BY-SA 3.0 <https://creativecommons.org/licenses/by-sa/3.0>, via Wikimedia Commons

Autosomal Recessive (AR)

Recessive conditions are expressed when an individual has *two copies of the mutant allele* (Figure 8.3).

Females and males are affected equally.

When an individual has just one copy of the mutant allele, they are said to be a 'carrier'.

Examples of AR include homocystinuria, phenylketonuria and Wilson's disease.

X-Linked Genetics

In sex-linked disorders, the mutated gene lies on the X chromosome. This means that *all males* are affected. Like autosomal conditions, these can be dominant or recessive.

Autosomal recessive

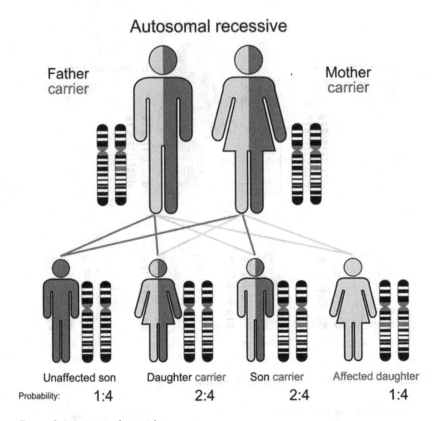

Figure 8.4 Autosomal recessive

Males inherit an X chromosome from their mother and a Y from their father, so affected *males are unable to pass the condition on to their sons.*

The inheritance pattern is characterised by transmission from affected males to male grandchildren via affected carrier daughters, known as the *Knight's move transmission.*

X-Linked Dominant

These conditions are *rare.*

The X chromosome must contain a disease-causing mutation; the most commonly used example is *vitamin D resistant rickets.*

A female with heterozygous XX or male XY will be affected.

Females are twice as likely to be affected, as they inherit two X chromosomes. If the affected male mates with a homozygous normal female, then all of the daughters will be affected but none of the sons.

Rett syndrome is X-linked and typically is only present in females.

Fragile X Syndrome

Fragile X syndrome is technically an X-linked dominant disorder. A mutated FMR1 gene could present with features of fragile X syndrome. However, it is *also a trinucleotide repeat disorder* and many people with the mutation will not have enough repeats to develop notable features of the disease.

X-Linked Recessive

Conversely, if a recessive disease-causing X chromosome is passed on to a male offspring, this is likely to cause a disease as there is no compensatory second X chromosome—whereas if it is passed on to a female offspring, an identical defect on the second X chromosome (extremely rare) would be necessary to cause the disease.

In comparison to dominant conditions, *skipped generations are common* because affected males can produce carrier daughters.

X-linked recessive disorders:

- Noonan syndrome
- Hurler syndrome
- Duchenne muscular dystrophy
- Red-green colour blindness
- Lesch-Nyhan syndrome
- Haemophilia A and B

h) Non-Mendelian Inheritance

Mitochondrial inheritance: all mitochondria in the sperm cell lies in its tail, which is shed on entry to the ovum, so all mitochondrial DNA is *inherited from the mother*.

Mitochondrial abnormalities can affect males and females.

Mitochondrial DNA contain *no introns*, so any mutations are likely to have an effect.

Mitochondrial mutations most commonly result in *myopathies* or *neuropathies*, such as Leber hereditary optic neuropathy, the most common cause of blindness in young men.

Trinucleotide repeats disorders are a set of genetic disorders caused by the presence of *additional sets of codons* repeating themselves in a specific gene.

The hallmark of these conditions is *anticipation*: a pattern of inheritance in which successive generations are affected at progressively *younger ages* and with *increasing severity*.

Important trinucleotide repeats disorders are outlined in Table 8.1:

Table 8.1 Trinucleotide repeats disorders

Condition	Repeat sequence involved
Friedreich's ataxia	GAA
Myotonic dystrophy	CTG
Spinocerebellar ataxia	CAG
Fragile X syndrome	CGG
Huntington's disease	CAG

i) Techniques in Molecular Genetics

Blotting techniques are methods of *detecting genetic material*, with different techniques used to detect different types of material:

- **Southern blotting**: used to detect specific *DNA sequences*
- **Northern blotting**: used to detect *RNA*
- **Western blotting**: used to detect *proteins*

Fluorescent in situ hybridisation (FISH) is used to identify *where* a particular gene falls within an individual's chromosomes.

A short sequence of single-stranded DNA is made that matches a portion of the gene the researcher is looking for. This piece of DNA is called a *probe* and attaches to a similar area on the chromosome with a fluorescent marker, allowing the researcher to identify its location.

j) Heritability

It is important to understand that heritability refers to the *population* rather than an individual. Heritability estimates how much *variation* in a phenotypic trait in a population is *due to genetic rather than environmental factors* among individuals in that population.

(Heritability is often misinterpreted as a measure of the extent to which genes are the cause of a disease.)

For example, some humans in a population are taller than others; heritability attempts to identify how much genetics play a role in part of the population being taller.

N.B., the **phenotype** is an organism's observable characteristics that result from a combination of gene expression and environmental factors.

If a condition has a heritability of 0.9, then 90% of the variance of that condition seen in a population is attributable to genetic variation. The remaining 10% is attributable to environmental factors.

Heritability of 0.0 indicates genes do not contribute at all to phenotypic differences in a population, whereas a heritability of 1 means genes account for all observed differences.

k) Concordance

Concordance is the probability that a pair of individuals will both have a certain trait, given that one of the pair has the trait. For example, twins are concordant for a disease when both have, or both lack, the given disease.

If the disease being studied has a significant genetic component, one would expect higher concordance in monozygotic (MZ) twins than dizygotic (DZ) twins.

If a trait has no genetic basis, it should have equivalent concordance rates in MZ and DZ twins.

l) Hardy–Weinberg Equilibrium

The law states that both allele and genotype frequencies in a population will remain constant from generation to generation, in a state of equilibrium, in the absence of other evolutionary influences.

Because one or more of these influences are typically present in real populations, the Hardy–Weinberg principle describes an ideal condition against which the effects of these influences can be analysed.

Evolutionary influences include:

- Mutations
- Gene flow—migration of individuals into and out of the population
- Genetic drift
- Natural selection
- Mate choice

m) Genetic Studies

Twin Studies

For discrete traits, resemblance is expressed in terms of *concordance* rates:

- A proband concordance rate is:

  the number of affected twins divided by the total number of co-twins.
  This method is more robust and allows for comparison with the general population.

- A **pairwise concordance rate** is:
  the number of twin pairs who both have the disease divided by the total number of pairs.

- A special type of twin study is to examine MZ twins reared apart.

Family Studies

- **Family history method** requires researchers to take a detailed history from the proband, which is then used to determine how many relatives are also affected.
- **Family study method** is a more robust method in which all the family members are interviewed.
- **Adoption studies** are used to differentiate the effects of the *environment vs. genetics*. They determine the rates of disease in biological relatives compared with adoptive relatives. Children that go through the adoption process might be more likely to develop psychiatric conditions, affecting the validity of these results.

n) Schizophrenia Genetics

Most common psychiatric disorders like schizophrenia do not show Mendelian genetics. It is commonly thought that these disorders are the result of *multifactorial inheritance*, a combination of genetic factors interacting jointly with environmental factors.

A number of studies have demonstrated a higher incidence of schizophrenia in first degree relatives of patients with the disease. It can be concluded that genetics play an important role in the development of schizophrenia.

The heritability of schizophrenia is *80%* (Onstad, 1991)[1]. Genetic concordance with other relatives is outlined in Table 8.2.

Schizophrenia is linked to a number of genes, and logic suggests that the more genes a person has, the greater risk that person has of developing schizophrenia.

Table 8.2 Genetic transmission of schizophrenia

Relationship to patient	Concordance
MZ twins	50%
DZ twins	17%
Parent	6%
Child	13%
Sibling	9%
Grandchild	5%

Table 8.3 Important genes identified in schizophrenia

Genes suspected	Locus
COMT (Catechol-O-Methyltransferase)	22q11
Dysbindin DTNBP1 (dystrobrevin binding protein 1)	6p22
NRG1 (Neuregulin)	8p12-p21
DISC1 (disrupted-in-schizophrenia 1)	1q42

Genes suspected to have a role in schizophrenia, as in Table 8.3.

Polygenic inheritance is again a complex inheritance pattern in which multiple genes are involved but *no environmental factors* are involved.

o) Affective Disorders Genetics

Bipolar Disorder

- Heritability is high: 85–90%.
- MZ twins: 40–70% concordance.
- First degree relatives: 5–10% concordance.
- General population: 0.5–1.5%.

Relatives of individuals with bipolar disorder are also more likely to develop a unipolar disorder.

Genes suspected to have a role in bipolar affective disorder are outlined in Table 8.4.

Unipolar Depression

- Heritability is unclear.
- General population: 5–10%.
- MZ twins: 40%.
- First degree relative: 5–30%.

p) Autism Genetics

- Heritability: 90%.
- Siblings of autistic individuals are approximately 50–100 times more likely to be born with autism than the general population.
- In MZ twins, the concordance is around 80–92%. In DZ twins, the concordance rate is 1–10%. This demonstrates the genetic complexity of these disorders.
- The identity and number of genes involved remains unknown. Chromosomes *2*, *7* and *15* are thought to be important.

Table 8.4 Importance genes identified in bipolar affective disorder

Genes suspected	Locus
COMT	22q11
DAO G72/G30	6p22
D amino oxidase	
BDNF (brain derived neurotrophic factor)	8p12-p21

- Autism is closely associated with single gene disorders. The most documented is fragile X.

  Sixteen percent of Fragile X males are autistic, whereas 8% of autistic children have fragile X.

q) Attention-Deficit/Hyperactivity Disorder (ADHD) Genetics

- Heritability: 70–80%.
- Risks are higher for male relatives.
- Risk to first degree relatives: 15–60%.
- Risk to second degree relatives: 3–9%.

r) Summary of Genetic Disorders

Table 8.5 provides a summary of genetic disorders that are relevant to psychiatry.

Table 8.5 Genetic disorders

Condition	Features	Chromosome
Down syndrome (trisomy 21)	• Almond-shaped eyes • Epicanthic folds • Simian crease • Short stature • Low-set ears • Brushfield spots Associated with mild to moderate learning disability (LD) and microcephaly, but not always.	21
Angelman syndrome (happy puppet syndrome)	• Flapping hands • Pronounced verbal delay compared with comprehension • Learning disability • Seizures • Disrupted sleep cycle	15q11 maternal origin

Condition	Features	Chromosome
Prader–Willi syndrome	• Hyperphagia • Obesity • Short stature • Small gonads • Hypotonia • Skin picking • Learning disability	15q11 paternal origin
Cri du chat	• 'Meow-like' cry • Hypertelorism • Microcephaly • Downturned mouth	5p deletion
Velocardiofacial syndrome (DiGeorge syndrome)	• Congenital cardiac disease • Cleft palate • Learning disability • Associated with high rates of psychosis compared to population	22q (deletion)
Edwards' syndrome (trisomy 18)	• Clubbed feet—rocker bottom • Webbed toes • Kidney malformations • Upturned nose	18
Lesch-Nyhan syndrome	• Self harm—head banging • Writhing movement • Dystonia	Xq26–27
Smith-Magenis syndrome	• Self-injurious behaviour	17p11
Fragile X	• Hand flapping • Elongated face • Large ears • Large testicles • Macrocephaly	X
Wolf-Hirschhorn syndrome	• Severe learning disability • Facial deformity • Seizures • Downturned mouth • Cleft palate	4p
Patau syndrome (trisomy 13)	• Learning disability • Polydactyl and overlapping of thumb and fingers • Microcephaly	13
Rett syndrome	• Affects girls exclusively • Symptoms start one year from birth • Regression and loss of skills • Hand wringing • Severe learning disability	Xq28
Tuberous sclerosis	• Tumours develop on various organs, including the brain • Associated with autism spectrum disorders (ASD)/ADHD and epilepsy	Genetically heterogeneous, linkage to 9q and 16p

(Continued)

Table 8.5 (Continued)

Condition	Features	Chromosome
Williams syndrome	• Sensitive hearing • Affinity for music • Friendly demeanour • Advanced verbal skills but superficial comprehension • Elf-like features	7q11 deletion
Rubinstein-Taybi syndrome	• Mild to moderate learning disability • Short stature • Small heads	Unclear; 16p deletions have been reported
Klinefelter syndrome	• Tall • Small gonads • Learning disability • Poor social skills	Extra X chromosome in phenotypic males (47 XXY)
Coffin–Lowry syndrome	• Slanted eyes • Big nose • Severe learning disability	Xp22
Turner syndrome	• Short stature • Webbed neck • Widely spaced nipples	45 X0
Niemann–Pick disease (types A and B)	• Cherry red spot • Abdominal swelling • Difficult to feed	11p15

Note

1. Onstad, S., I. Skre, S. Torgersen, & E. Kringlen. (1991). Twin concordance for DSM-III-R schizophrenia. *Acta Psychiatrica Scandinavica*, 83 (5): 395–401.

Source Material

Blakemore, S.-J., and U. Frith. (2005). *The Learning Brain*. Victoria, Australia: Blackwell Publishing.

Franke, B., S. V. Faraone, P. Asherson, J. Buitelaar, C. H. Bau, J. A. Ramos-Quiroga, E. Mick, E. H. Grevet, S. Johansson, J. Haavik, K. P. Lesch, B. Cormand, and A. Reif. (October 2012). The Genetics of Attention Deficit/Hyperactivity Disorder in Adults: A Review. *Molecular Psychiatry*, 17 (10): 960–987.

Kumar, Parveen, and Michael L. Clark. (2016). *Kumar and Clark's Clinical Medicine*. London: Elsevier, 9th ed., pp. 0–1456.

Nolen-Hoeksema, S. (2013). *Abnormal Psychology*. New York, 6th ed., p. 267.

Nolen-Hoeksema, S. (2014). Neurodevelopmental and Neurocognitive Disorders. In *Abnormal Psychology*. New York: McGraw-Hill, 6th ed.

Penfield, W., and T. Rasmussen. (1950). *The Cerebral Cortex of a Man: A Clinical Study of Localization of Function*. New York: Palgrave Macmillan.

Strachan, Tom, and Andrew Read. (2010). *Human Molecular Genetics*. London: Garland Science, 4th ed., pp. 0–808.

Sullivan, P. F., M. C. Neale, and K. S. Kendler. (2000). Genetic Epidemiology of Major Depression: Review and Meta-Analysis. *American Journal of Psychiatry*, 157: 1552–1562.

Tatum, William O. (2014). *Handbook of EEG Interpretation*. New York: Demos Medical Publishing, pp. 155–190.

Tortora, Gerard J., and Bryan H. Derrickson. (2014). *Principles of Anatomy and Physiology*. London: John Wiley & Sons, pp. 0–1300.

9   Clinical Neuropathology

Elizabeth Templeton

a) Alzheimer's Disease (AD)

Macroscopic Neuropathology

- Diffuse atrophy (most marked in the frontal and temporal lobes)
- Flattened cortical sulci
- Enlarged cerebral ventricles

Histological Changes/Microscopic

(Remember *plaques*, *tangles* and *hirano bodies*.)

- Neuronal loss (particularly in the cortex and the hippocampus)
- Shrinking of dendritic branches
- Reactive astrocytosis

Changes commonly seen in the hippocampus include:

- Neuritic senile plaques—insoluble *amyloid* peptide deposits
- Neurofibrillary tangles (NFTs)—primarily abnormally phosphorylated *tau protein*
- Granulovacuolar degeneration
- Hirano bodies

AD is one of several 'degenerative tauopathies'.
   Tau is a peptide required for *microtubule synthesis*.
   Microtubules allow for transport of materials down the axons.
   The number and distribution of tangles *correlates* to the degree of cognitive decline.
   Granulovacuolar degeneration: small vacuoles containing central granules in the cytoplasm of neurons.
   Hirano body: intracellular aggregates of actin and actin-associated proteins. These are seen in the extracellular space when neurons die, frequently in *pyramidal cells* of the *hippocampus*.

DOI: 10.1201/9781003322573-13

Astrocytosis: an abnormal increase in the number of astrocytes due to the destruction of nearby neurons from CNS trauma (also known as astrogliosis or referred to as reactive astrocytosis).

Binswanger's Disease—White Matter Disease

This is also known as *subcortical* vascular dementia or subcortical arteriosclerotic encephalopathy.

It is characterised by the presence of small *infarctions of the white matter* that *spares cortical regions*.

---

b) Lewy Body Dementia (LBD)

(Remember *Lewy bodies*.)
   Histological changes:

* **Lewy bodies**: weakly eosinophilic spherical cytoplasmic inclusions
* Neuronal loss
* Neuritic senile plaques
* NFTs

Lewy bodies are also found in Parkinson's disease within the substantia nigra. However, in LBD, the density and distribution of Lewy bodies is much greater, particularly in the cingulate gyrus, parahippocampal gyrus and temporal cortex.

Lewy bodies in the substantia nigra have a clear halo, which can be used to differentiate them from cortical Lewy bodies.

There is *no correlation* between number of Lewy bodies and cognitive decline.

Lewy bodies contain accumulations of *alpha synuclein*, which accelerate the reuptake of dopamine in neurons, creating a toxic overload of dopamine in the cortex.

LBD is one of the *synucleopathies*.

c) Frontotemporal Dementia (FTD)

FTD is associated with three types of underlying pathology: frontal lobe degeneration, Pick's disease and motor neuron disease (MND).

The exam questions focus mainly on Pick's disease.

Pick's Disease

Macroscopic changes:

* Selective *asymmetrical* atrophy in the frontal and anterior temporal region

- *Knife blade gyri*
- Ventricular enlargement

Histological changes predominantly seen in the cerebral cortex basal ganglia, locus coeruleus and sunstantia nigra:

- Loss of large cortical nerve cells
- Reactive astrocytosis
- Pick bodies
- Pick cells (balloon cells)

Pick bodies are composed of randomly arranged *filaments of tau* protein.
  Hirano bodies may also be seen but with lesser frequency than in AD.

d) Creutzfeldt-Jakob Disease (CJD)

Three types of CJD exist: sporadic (most common), familial and variant CJD (vCJD, related to bovine spongiform encephalopathy).
  Individuals with the disease often have a poor prognosis and die within the first 6–12 months. As a result, there are limited gross pathological features.

Macroscopic changes:

- Generalised cerebral atrophy
- Selective cerebellar atrophy
- Ventricular enlargement

Histological changes:

- Neuronal loss
- *Spongiform encephalopathy*—many oval vacuoles are seen in the neutrophils of cortical grey matter
- Astrocytic proliferation

CJD is transmitted by infection with an abnormal prion protein (PrP).
  Infection might be transmitted from contaminated electrodes after neurosurgical procedures, corneal transplants or pituitary extracts.
  MRI is the most useful diagnostic test in variant CJD: the *pulvinar sign* is a characteristic abnormality seen in the *posterior thalamic region* and is highly sensitive and specific for variant CJD.
  Pulvinar symmetrical hyperintensity are seen in the pulvinar (posterior) nuclei of the thalamus (Figure 9.1).

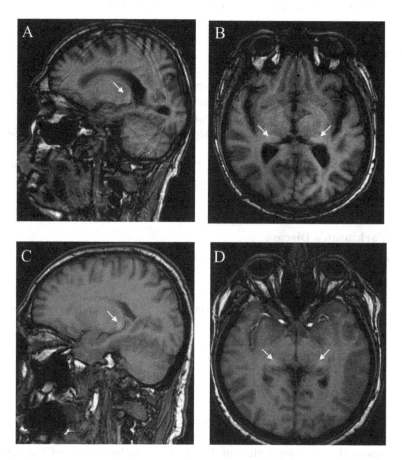

Figure 9.1 MRI showing pulvinar sign

e) Schizophrenia

Gross neuropathology:

- Decrease in brain weight, length and volume.
- A reduction in the volume of cerebral hemispheres, cortex and grey matter.
- Ventricular enlargement.
- Post-mortem studies have shown reduced volume in the temporal lobe, particularly affecting the grey matter, amygdala and anterior hippocampus.

- Increased incidence of *cavum septi pellucidi* is noted.
- Consistent *reversal of the planum temporale.*

Histological changes:

- Increase in neuronal density, perhaps due to a reduction in neuronal size.
- Reduced cell size and numbers, particularly in the *dorsolateral prefrontal cortex* (DLPFC) and the *hippocampus.*
- Cytoarchitectural abnormalities in the entorhinal cortex such as disruption of the cortical layers.
- Decrease in pre-synaptic markers. These changes could reflect a reduction in synaptic contacts and support the theory of *excessive synaptic pruning* in schizophrenia.

f) Parkinson's Disease

Macroscopic changes:

- Diffuse cortical atrophy.
- *Depigmentation* in the locus coeruleus and substantia nigra (zona compacta).

Histological changes:

- Neuronal loss.
- Reactive astrocytosis.
- Lewy bodies are present in the cerebral cortex, limbic system and in many extra-nigral, nondopaminergic neuronal groups, including the locus coeruleus, dorsal motor nucleus of the vagus, the nucleus basalis of Meynert, sympathetic ganglia and myenteric plexus.

g) Summary of Pathological Findings

Table 9.1 provides a summary of pathological findings that are relevant to psychiatry.

Table 9.1 Pathological findings

Pathology	Disease
Asteroid bodies	Sarcoidosis and berylliosis
Barr bodies	Stains of X chromosomes
Hirano bodies	Normal aging, but more numerous in Alzheimer's disease
Kayser—Fleischer rings	Wilson's disease

Pathology	Disease
Knife blade gyri	Pick's disease
Kuru plaques	Kuru and Gerstmann-Sträussler syndrome, and are sometimes present in patients with Creutzfeldt-Jakob disease (CJD)
LE bodies (a.k.a hematoxylin bodies)	Systemic lupus erythematosus (SLE) (lupus)
Lewy bodies	Parkinson's disease and Lewy body dementia
Mallory bodies	Found in alcoholic hepatitis, alcoholic cirrhosis, Wilson's disease and primary-biliary cirrhosis
Neurofibrillary tangles	Alzheimer's disease
Pick bodies	Frontotemporal dementia
Pulvinar sign	Creutzfeldt-Jakob disease
Schaumann bodies	Sarcoidosis and berylliosis
Verocay bodies	Schwannoma (neurilemoma)
Zebra bodies	Niemann-Pick disease, Tay-Sachs disease, or any of the mucopolysaccharidoses

Source Material

Cain, H., and B. Kraus. (1983). Immunofluorescence Microscopic Demonstration of Vimentin Filaments in Asteroid Bodies of Sarcoidosis: A Comparison with Electron Microscopic Findings. *Virchows Archive B Cell Pathology Including Molecular Pathology*, 42 (2): 213–226.

Dimitri, P., and M. D. Agamanolis. (2015). *Neuropathology – An Interactive Course for Medical Students and Residents* [ONLINE]. Available at: http://neuropathology-web.org/chapter10/chapter10bLSDs.html. [Accessed September 25, 2017].

Esiri, Margaret M., James H. Morris, John Q. Trojanowski, and Virginia M. Y. Lee. (2004). *The Neuropathology of Dementia*. Cambridge: Cambridge University Press, pp. 0–584.

Jensen, K., and C. Gluud. (October 1994). The Mallory Body: Morphological, Clinical and Experimental Studies (Part 1 of a Literature Survey). *Hepatology*, 20 (4 Pt 1): 1061–1077.

Kendler, K. S., M. McGuire, A. M. Gruenberg, A. Ohare, M. Spellman, and D. Walsh. (1993). The Roscommon Family Study. 1. Methods, Diagnosis of Probands, and Risk of Schizophrenia in Relatives. *Archives of General Psychiatry*, 50: 527–540.

Kumar, Parveen, and Michael L. Clark. (2016). *Kumar and Clark's Clinical Medicine*. London: Elsevier, 9th ed., pp. 0–1456.

Strachan, Tom, and Andrew Read. (2010). *Human Molecular Genetics*. London: Garland Science, 4th ed., pp. 0–808.

10 Applied Neurosciences

Elizabeth Templeton

a) Frontal Lobe

Tests of the frontal lobe are explained in Table 10.1.

Generally, **damage to the frontal lobes** causes problems with 'executive function', the ability to plan and initiate movement, such as crossing the street or answering complex questions.

Anterior Frontal Lobe Lesions

* Striking *loss of inhibition*—subjects might become inappropriately elevated and euphoric or depressed
* Abulia: lack of decisiveness and drive
* Loss of verbal fluency
* Apathy
* Difficulty processing and retaining information

Medial Frontal Lobe (Broca's Area) Lesions

* *Expressive aphasia* (broken speech)

Anterior Frontal Lobe Lesions

* The frontal lobe controls voluntary movement; damage to this area can cause *contralateral hemiparesis*

b) Parietal Lobe

Functions of the parietal lobe are explained in Table 10.2.

c) Temporal Lobe Lesions

The left temporal lobe (usually the dominant side in right-handed people) is responsible for *language comprehension*.

DOI: 10.1201/9781003322573-14

Table 10.1 Tests of the frontal lobe

Test	Explanation
Abstract thinking	Proverb interpretation: *'people in glass houses should not throw stones'.* Similarities: *'what are the similarities between apples and grapes?—they are both fruits'.*
Motor sequencing	Luria three-step tests; ask the patient to copy your actions: fist, palm, edge. Do not give verbal prompts.
Inhibition	Go/no go test: ask the patient to raise their hand when you tap once and not to raise it when you tap twice.
Cognitive estimates	*'What is the height of the average English woman?'* *'What is the best-paying job in Britain?'*
Trail making test	Test A: uses a number sequence to join the dots. Test B: thought to be more sensitive, using an alternate number or letter sequence to join the dots.
Primitive reflexes	Stroke the patient's thenar eminence. A positive result would be the patient wincing.

Table 10.2 Parietal lobe functions

Test	Explanation
Agraphia	Inability to communicate in writing.
Graphesthesia	Inability to recognise writing on the skin by touch alone.
Stereognosis	Inability to identify items through touch, such as a coin or pen.
Two-point discrimination	Distinguish whether two points touching the skin are truly separate or a single point. Relevant to cortical sensation.
Right-left disorientation	Ask the patient to close their eyes and touch their left ear with their right hand.
Finger agnosia	Ask patient to close their eyes and identify the finger that is being touched.
Hemi-neglect	Ask the patient to draw a person. A positive result occurs if the patient only draws one side.
Apraxia	Dressing: ask the patient to do up buttons on their shirt. Constructional apraxia: ask the patient to copy interlocking pentagons.

Damage there can cause **Wernicke's aphasia**: speech production is normal, but comprehension is impaired.

If the right temporal lobe is damaged, people might have impaired auditory verbal learning or inability to sing.

Temporal Lobe Epilepsy (TLE)

Seizures are commonly associated with auras, the most common causing an epigastric sensation.

Geschwind syndrome: rarely, temporal lobe seizure can produce a type of personality change. An individual may become humourless, obsessive, pre-occupied with religion or increasingly promiscuous.

Occipital Lobe Lesions

Bilateral damage to the occipital lobe results in *cortical blindness*.

Unilateral lesions can result in *contralateral* central or peripheral *homonymous hemianopia*.

Visual illusions and hallucinations are associated with *right* sided occipital lesions.

Text Box 10.1

Anton-Babinski Syndrome

Anton-Babinski syndrome, or visual anosognosia, is rare symptom of brain damage occurring in the occipital lobe.

Patients experience cortical blindness but lack insight and often deny their blindness, despite clear evidence to the contrary. Confabulation often occurs in order to make up for the loss of sensory input.

---

d) Apraxia

Apraxia is a neurological movement disorder caused by damage to the *posterior parietal lobe*.

Individuals struggle to perform learned voluntary movements when requested. The main types of functional apraxia are summarised in Table 10.3.

Table 10.3 Main types of functional apraxia

Limb kinetic apraxia	Loss of hand and finger dexterity leads to an inability to make fine or delicate movements.
Constructional apraxia	Inability to copy a picture or combine parts of something to make a whole.
Ideational apraxia	Inability to carry out a sequence of actions to complete a task; *'fold a piece of paper in half and put it under the chair'*. Here the patient does not know 'what' to do.
Ideomotor apraxia (most common)	*Impairment of goal-directed movement.* The patient cannot complete learned tasks when give the correct equipment, for example, if given a hairbrush, the patient knows what to do but not 'how' to do it.
Buccofacial apraxia	Inability to control lip and facial muscles such as when winking, whistling and coughing on demand.
Oculomotor	Inability to control eye movements.

e) Language

Aphasia refers to an inability to use or understand language despite intact hearing and sound production.

Aphasia is an acquired disorder, causes of which are outlined in Table 10.4. It does not include developmental conditions, thought disorder or purely motor impairments such as stammering.

Language Production Model

Sound:

*   Wernicke's area + auditory association cortex for processing
*   Via arcuate fasciculus, connects Wernicke's and Broca's areas
*   Signals from Broca's area are relied to the motor area
*   Movement of tongue, lips and vocal cords

f) Agnosia

Agnosia refers to the *inability to recognise* objects, people, sounds or smells whilst the relative sense remains intact, as outlined in Table 10.5.

Table 10.4 Aphasias

Wernicke's aphasia (jargon aphasia)	This occurs due to a lesion in Wernicke's area, the *posterior region of the superior temporal gyrus*. The *comprehension* of language is impaired. The speech production is *fluent but meaningless*. It may mimic thought disorder.
Broca's aphasia	This occurs following damage to the Broca's area (Brodmann areas *44* and *45*) in the frontal lobe. Speech is broken/*non-fluent* and can appear laboured, with frequent pauses.
Conduction aphasia	Damage to the *arcuate fasciculus*. Speech is *fluent* and *comprehension is intact*. *Repetition and naming are impaired*.
Anomic aphasia	The lesions are often *temporal/parietal*. Patients present with *naming or word finding difficulty*. Repetition and comprehension are intact.

Table 10.5 Agnosias

Anosognosia	Inability to recognise own condition/illness.
Autotopagnosia	Inability to orient parts of the body.
Phonagnosia	Inability to recognise familiar voices.
Simultanagnosia	Inability to appreciate two objects in the visual field at the same time.
Astereoagnosia	Inability to recognise objects by touch.
Prosopagnosia	Inability to recognise a familiar face.

Source Material

Alexander, M. P., and A. E. Hillis. (2008). In Georg Goldenberg, Bruce L. Miller, Michael J. Aminoff, Francois Boller, D. F. Swaab (Eds.), *Aphasia: Handbook of Clinical Neurology*. Amsterdam: Elsevier, 1st ed., Vol. 88, pp. 287–310.

Blakemore, S-J., and U. Frith. (2005). *The Learning Brain*. Victoria: Blackwell Publishing.

Burns, M. S. (2004). Clinical Management of Agnosia. *Topics in Stroke Rehabilitation*, 11 (1): 1–9.

Davis, Larry E., and Sarah Pirio Richardson. (2015–2005–2029). *Fundamentals of Neurologic Disease*. New York: Springer, p. 139.

Kumar, Parveen, and Michael L. Clark. (2016). *Kumar and Clark's Clinical Medicine*. London: Elsevier, 9th ed., pp. 0–1456.

Nolen-Hoeksema, S. (2014). Neurodevelopmental and Neurocognitive Disorders. In *Abnormal Psychology*. New York: McGraw-Hill, 6th ed.

Penfield, W., and T. Rasmussen. (1950). *The Cerebral Cortex of a Man: A Clinical Study of Localization of Function*. New York: Palgrave Macmillan.

Sathian, K., L. J. Buxbaum, L. G. Cohen, J. W. Krakauer, C. E. Lang, M. Corbetta, and S. M. Fitzpatrick. (June 2011). Neurological and Rehabilitation of Action Disorders: Common Clinica Deficits. *Neurorehabilitation and Neural Repair*, 25 (5): 21S–32S.

Part IV

Clinical Psychopharmacology

11 Mechanisms of Psychotropic Drugs

Lisanne Stock

a) Classification of Psychotropic Medications

Drugs which affect a person's mood, thoughts or perceptions are known as psychotropic drugs and these can be in the form of prescribed or recreational drugs.

The main classes of drugs used in psychiatry are:

- Antipsychotics
- Antidepressants
- Anxiolytics
- Antiepileptics
- Mood stabilisers
- Drugs used in the treatment of dementia
- Drugs used in the treatment of attention-deficit/hyperactivity disorder (ADHD)
- Drugs used in the treatment of substance misuse

The main classes of recreational drug include:

- Psychostimulants
- Cannabinoids
- Hallucinogenics
- Novel psychoactive substances

Non-psychotropic medications are also often used by patients with a psychiatric background, and some examples are discussed later in the chapter.

b) Typical Antipsychotics

Typical (first generation) antipsychotics (Table 11.1) are highly associated with extrapyramidal side effects (EPSEs) and raised prolactin levels. With long-term use they can lead to tardive dyskinesia, a disorder of involuntary movements which can be difficult to reverse.

DOI: 10.1201/9781003322573-16

Table 11.1 Typical antipsychotics

Chlorpromazine	Chlorpromazine is a phenothiazine antipsychotic. It acts as an antagonist of D1, D2, D3 and D4 dopaminergic receptors and 5HT1 and 5HT2 serotonergic receptors.
Haloperidol	Haloperidol is an antagonist of D2 dopamine receptors.
Sulpiride	Sulpiride is a selective antagonist of D2 dopamine receptor.
Trifluoperazine	Trifluoperazine is an antagonist of D1 and D2 dopaminergic receptors.

c) Atypical Antipsychotics

Atypical/second generation antipsychotics (Table 11.2) are associated with fewer EPSEs but more metabolic side effects such as weight gain and dyslipidaemia.

Table 11.2 Atypical antipsychotics

Amisulpride	Amisulpride is a *D2* and *D3* dopamine receptor antagonist.
Aripiprazole	Aripiprazole is a *D2* dopamine receptor and *5HT1A* serotonin receptor partial agonist. It also works as an antagonist at α-adrenergic and *5HT2A* serotonin receptors.
Lurasidone	Lurasidone is a *D2* dopamine receptor, *5-HT2A* serotonin receptor, *α2A* and *α2C*-adrenergic receptor antagonist.
Olanzapine	Olanzapine is a *D1, D2, D3* and *D4* dopaminergic receptor antagonist. It is also an antagonist at *5HT2A, 5HT2C, 5HT3* and *5HT6* serotonin receptors, *α1*-adrenergic receptors, *H1* histamine receptors and multiple muscarinic receptors.
Quetiapine	Quetiapine is a *D1* and *D2* dopamine receptor antagonist and *5HT2A* serotonin receptor antagonist.
Risperidone	Risperidone is a *D2* dopamine receptor antagonist and *5HT2A* serotonin receptor antagonist. It is also an *H1* histamine receptor antagonist.
Clozapine	Clozapine is a *D1* and *D2* dopamine receptor antagonist and *5HT2A* serotonin receptor antagonist.

d) Antidepressants

Table 11.3 describes the mechanism of action for different classes of antidepressants.

Table 11.3 Mechanism of action of antidepressants

Selective serotonin reuptake inhibitors (SSRIs)	SSRIs inhibit the presynaptic reuptake of the neurotransmitter *serotonin* via the serotonin transporter, therefore increasing the amount of serotonin in the synapse and consequently its effects within the brain. Examples: sertraline, fluoxetine, citalopram and paroxetine

Tricyclic antidepressants (TCAs)	TCAs inhibit the re-uptake of *noradrenaline* via the noradrenaline transporter and *serotonin* via the serotonin transporter. These are sodium dependent membrane pumps and via reducing the re-uptake of these neurotransmitters, they increase their concentration at the synaptic clefts of the neural connections within the brain. Examples: amitriptyline and imipramine
Monoamine oxidase inhibitors (MAOIs)	MAOIs inhibit the action of the enzyme *monoamine oxidase*. They are not commonly used due to multiple drug interactions as well as interactions with tyramine containing foods for example cheese (*see Text box* 12.2). Examples: moclobemide (selective, reversible inhibition of MAO-A) and selegiline (selective, irreversible inhibition of MAO-B)
Noradrenaline and specific serotonergic *antidepressants* (*NASSAs*)	NASSAs act as antagonists of *5HT2* and *5HT3* serotonin receptors and also act as peripheral *α1* and *α2*-adrenergic receptor antagonists. They also act as *H1* histamine receptor inverse agonists. Examples: mirtazapine and mianserin
Noradrenaline reuptake inhibitors (NaRI)	NaRIs inhibit *noradrenaline* re-uptake by blocking the noradrenaline transporter leading to increased levels of extracellular adrenaline and noradrenaline. Examples: reboxetine and atomoxetine
Serotonin norepinephrine reuptake inhibitor (SNRIs)	SNRIs inhibit the reuptake of *serotonin* and *noradrenaline* via selective inhibition of serotonin and noradrenaline transporters. They also have an inhibitory effect on the dopamine transporter but to a lesser extent. Examples: venlafaxine and duloxetine
Melatonergic agonists	Melatonergic agonists act as agonists at *MT1* and *MT2* melatonin receptors. Examples: melatonin and agomelatine

e) Anxiolytics and Sedatives

Table 11.4 describes the mechanism of action for different classes of anxiolytics and sedatives.

Table 11.4 Mechanism of action of anxiolytics and sedatives

Benzodiazepines	Benzodiazepines act as *GABA-A* receptor agonists, enhancing GABA transmission in the central nervous system via the opening of chloride ion channels, increasing the inhibitory effect of GABA. Examples: lorazepam (short acting benzodiazepine) and clonazepam (intermediate-acting benzodiazepine)
Z drugs	Z drugs are non-benzodiazepine hypnotics used for short-term management of insomnia. They bind to the same binding site on *GABA-A* receptors as the benzodiazepine subtype where they have an agonist effect via the same mechanism. Examples: zopiclone and zolpidem

(*Continued*)

Table 11.4 (Continued)

Melatonin	**Melatonin** is an endogenous hormone produced by the pineal gland that regulates sleep-wake cycles. It acts as an agonist at *MT1* and *MT2* melatonin receptors.
Promethazine	Promethazine is a first-generation antihistamine with sedative properties and acts primarily as an antagonist of *H1* histamine receptors but also as an antagonist at *α-adrenergic*, *anticholinergic* and *5HT2* serotonin receptors.

f) Antiepileptics and Mood Stabilisers

Table 11.5 describes the mechanism of action for different classes of antiepileptics and mood stabilisers.

Table 11.5 Mechanism of action of antiepileptics and mood stabilisers

Lithium	Lithium reduces excitatory neurotransmitters, *dopamine* and *glutamate* and increases inhibitory *GABA* levels in the brain via a number of neuro-chemical cascades.
Sodium valproate	Sodium valproate is thought to block *voltage-gated sodium channels* and inhibits *GABA* transaminase, leading to increased levels of GABA in the synaptic clefts within the brain.
Lamotrigine	Lamotrigine blocks *sodium channels* which inhibit the release of excitatory neurotransmitters *glutamate* and *aspartate*.
Vigabatrin	Vigabatrin inhibits *GABA* transaminase leading to increased levels of GABA in the brain.
Gabapentin	Gabapentin binds to the α2- δ subunit of voltage gated calcium channels and reduces release of *glutamate*.
Carbamazepine	Carbamazepine blocks *voltage-gated sodium channels*.

g) Dementia Drugs

Table 11.6 describes the mechanism of action for dementia drugs.

Table 11.6 Dementia drugs

Donepezil	Donepezil is an *acetylcholinesterase* inhibitor.
Rivastigmine	Rivastigmine is an *acetylcholinesterase* and *butyrylcholinesterase* inhibitor.
Galantamine	Galantamine is an *acetylcholinesterase* inhibitor.
Memantine	Memantine is an *NMDA* receptor antagonist.

h) ADHD Drugs

Table 11.7 describes the mechanism of action for AHDH drugs.

i) Drugs Used in the Treatment of Substance Misuse

Table 11.8 describes the mechanism of action for drugs used in the treatment of substance misuse.

Table 11.7 ADHD drugs

Methylphenidate	Methylphenidate is a *noradrenaline* and *dopamine* reuptake inhibitor (NDRI).
Lisdexamfetamine	Lisdexamfetamine is a prodrug of dextroamphetamine. The active form of this drug blocks the reuptake of *noradrenaline* and *dopamine* into the presynaptic neuron and increases their release into the synaptic cleft.
Atomoxetine	Atomoxetine is a *serotonin noradrenaline* reuptake inhibitor.
Clonidine	Clonidine is a *α2-adrenergic* receptor agonist.
Modafinil	Modafinil is a stimulant that acts as a *dopamine* reuptake inhibitor leading to an increase in dopamine levels.
Guanfacine	Guanfacine is an *α2-adrenergic* receptor agonist.

Table 11.8 Drugs used in the treatment of substance misuse

Bupropion	Bupropion is a *noradrenaline-dopamine* re-uptake inhibitor used to aid smoking cessation.
Methadone	Methadone is an opioid analgesic which acts as an agonist at the *μ-opioid* receptor and is used as a maintenance treatment for opioid dependence.
Naloxone	Naloxone is a competitive antagonist of the *μ-opioid* receptor, and it is used in the rapid reversal of opioid toxicity.
Suboxone	Suboxone is a combination of buprenorphine and naloxone and is used to reduce withdrawal symptoms in opioid dependence.
Naltrexone	Naltrexone is a competitive antagonist at the *μ-opioid κ-opioid* and *δ-opioid* receptors used to reduce cravings and withdrawal symptoms in opioid dependence.
Buprenorphine·	Buprenorphine is a partial agonist at the *μ-opioid* receptor and a *κ-opioid* receptor antagonist. It is an *α2-adrenergic* receptor agonist. It is used to reduce withdrawal symptoms in opioid dependence.
Lofexidine	Lofexidine is an *α2-adrenergic* agonist used to reduce cravings and withdrawal symptoms in opioid dependence.

j) Recreational Drugs[1,2]

Table 11.9 outlines the effect of commonly used recreational drugs.

Table 11.9 Recreational drugs

Psychostimulants	Enhance transmission at catecholaminergic synapses increasing *adrenaline*, *noradrenaline* and *dopamine* release. Examples: cocaine and methamphetamine (ecstasy)
Sedatives	Sedatives are taken to induce a feeling of relaxation, reduce irritability and in some cases pain relief or sleep. Examples: opioids, barbiturates and benzodiazepines Opioids are agonists at opioid receptors. Examples: morphine and diamorphine (heroin), which both act at *μ -opioid* agonists

(Continued)

Table 11.9 (Continued)

	Barbiturates: *GABA-A* receptor agonists. Examples: phenobarbital and barbital Benzodiazepines are *GABA-A* receptor agonists. Examples: lorazepam and clonazepam
Cannabinoids	Cannabinoids can be classified both as sedatives and as hallucinogens. Cannabis is made up of two main active compounds, *tetrahydrocannabinol* (THC) and *cannabidiol* (CBD), which have different receptor activities. Broadly, both act as *cannabinoid* receptor agonists. Spice is a synthetic cannabinoid which also acts as a cannabinoid receptor agonist.
Hallucinogens	Hallucinogens are associated with perceptual abnormalities in all modalities including visual, auditory, gustatory and olfactory hallucinations. They are also associated with euphoria, disinhibition and detachment from reality. Phencyclidine (PCP or angel dust) and ketamine: *NMDA* receptor antagonist. LSD (lysergic acid diethylamide): *5HT* receptor agonist. GHB (γ hydroxybutyrate): *GABA-B* and *GHB* receptor agonist.

Notes

1. [Online] https://go.drugbank.com/drugs/.
2. Enevoldson, T P. (2004). Recreational drugs and their neurological consequences. BMJ Journal of Neurology, Neurosurgery and Psychiatry, 75 (3).

12 Specifics of Prescribing

Lisanne Stock

a) Rational Prescribing

Rational prescribing refers to prescribing with a patient in mind and thinking about:

- The individual and their values, goals and aspirations.
- The diagnosis and other co-morbidities.
- Previous medications trialled and the outcomes of these.
- Long-term effects, including side effects and personalised life impact.
- Prognosis.

Risk and benefit appraisal refers to a prescriber thinking carefully about the pros and cons of a medication for an individual, taking into account all of the features of rational prescribing.

Prescribing in psychiatry is becoming increasingly personalised and rational prescribing allows a less formulaic approach to medication choice.

Advances in modern medicine have allowed for the type of medication to be chosen for a patient based on their genetic makeup. In some cases, clinicians are able to choose a drug tailored around the patient's likely response based on specific genes they might have and their genetic makeup as a whole (pharmacogenomics and pharmacogenetics).

b) Drugs With Psychiatric Side Effects[1]

There are a number of non-psychotropic drugs that are associated with changes in mental state. Table 12.1 shows some of the major groups of drugs and their associated psychiatric effects.

DOI: 10.1201/9781003322573-17

Text Box 12.1

Carbamazepine is an example of a medication where pharmacogenomics can be put into practice. Carbamazepine is associated with hypersensitivity reactions in up to 10% of patients, including severe reactions such as Steven-Johnson syndrome and toxic epidermal necrolysis. The risk of hypersensitivity is increased by the presence of certain human leucocyte antigens (HLA) alleles such as HLA B*15:02. This allele is present commonly in Southeast Asia (up to 15% of the population have HLA B*15:02 in Hong Kong) and guidelines recommend conducting genomic testing prior to prescribing carbamazepine in this population.[2]

Table 12.1 Drugs with psychiatric side effects

Steroids	Anabolic steroids as well as medically prescribed steroids can lead to *irritability*, *depression*, *anxiety* and in some cases induce a psychotic state.
Anti-epileptics	Anti-epileptics can lead to *irritability* and *agitation* and in some cases depression. Mood stabilising anti-epileptics are used in the treatment of bipolar disorder specifically for their effect on mental state and management of manic presentations.
Analgesics	Opioid analgesics are *addictive* and are associated with recreational drug abuse due to their euphoric effects. They can also cause *confusion* and *drowsiness*.
Anticholinergics	Anticholinergics can lead to *sedation*, *confusion* and *depression*, especially in elderly patients. In rare cases they have been associated with visual and auditory hallucinations.
Beta blockers	Beta blockers such as propranolol can be prescribed to help with anxiety. *Confusion* and *fatigue* are common side effects and rarely they can lead to hallucinations.
Dopaminergic agonists	Dopaminergic agonists can lead to *confusion*, *insomnia*, *hallucinations* and *impulse control* disorders.
Antimalarials	Antimalarials can lead to *vivid dreams*, *insomnia*, *anxiety*, *irritability*, *confusion* and *depression*.
Antihistaminergic	Some antihistaminergic medications can be *sedating* and medications such as promethazine are used specifically for this effect. Cyclizine when given intravenously is associated with euphoria and addiction.
Thyroid medications	Levothyroxine is associated with *anxiety* and *insomnia*.
Antibiotics	Quinolones such as ciprofloxacin are associated with *agitation*, *disorientation*, *anxiety* and *memory impairment* and rarely can induce a psychotic disorder. Metronidazole can lead to confusion and has in rare situations been associated with psychosis.

c) Side Effects of Antidepressants[3,4]

Each class of antidepressants is associated with distinct groups of side effects, but broadly, these can be recalled with the mnemonic GRAINS:

- Gastro-intestinal bleeding
- Rashes
- Antimuscarinic effects, for example, dry mouth and constipation
- Increased anxiety
- Nausea
- Sexual problems including reduced libido, anorgasmia and impotence

Rarer side effects include (ssssh!):

- Suicidal thoughts, particularly in the first few weeks
- Syndrome of inappropriate antidiuretic hormone secretion (SIADH)
- Serotonin syndrome
- Seizures
- Hyperprolactinemia and associated galactorrhoea

Text Box 12.2

A note on MAOIs: A tyramine induced MAOI reaction also known as the *cheese reaction* can lead to a hypertensive crisis if patients taking a MAOI has food and drink with high levels of tyramine including cheese, broad beans, chocolate and beer.[5] They are also associated with multiple drug interactions and withdrawal effects and for this reason are not commonly used in clinical practice.

---

d) Antidepressant Withdrawal

When a patient is started on antidepressants, they need to be informed of the potential for withdrawal symptoms upon discontinuation. Discontinuation symptoms usually occur within five days of stopping the antidepressant.

Antidepressants with a shorter half-life are associated more commonly with withdrawal symptoms and these include *paroxetine, venlafaxine* and *imipramine.* (1)

Common symptoms of antidepressant withdrawal include the following, which can be remembered using the mnemonic FACES:

- Flu-like symptoms, including myalgia, nausea, headache and sweating
- Agitation and irritability
- Concentration difficulties
- Electric shock-like sensations and other sensory disturbances

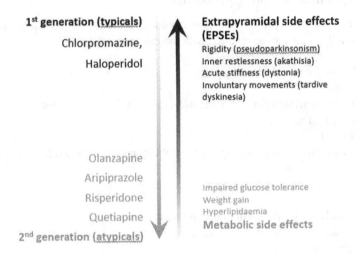

1ˢᵗ generation (typicals)
Chlorpromazine,
Haloperidol

Extrapyramidal side effects (EPSEs)
Rigidity (pseudoparkinsonism)
Inner restlessness (akathisia)
Acute stiffness (dystonia)
Involuntary movements (tardive dyskinesia)

Olanzapine
Aripiprazole
Risperidone
Quetiapine
2ⁿᵈ generation (atypicals)

Impaired glucose tolerance
Weight gain
Hyperlipidaemia
Metabolic side effects

Figure 12.1 Side effects of antipsychotics

Table 12.2 Side effects of antipsychotics

	Haloperidol	Aripiprazole	Olanzapine	Risperidone	Clozapine
Extrapyramidal effects	High	Rare	Mild	Moderate	Rare
Postural hypotension	Low	Mild	Mild	Moderate	High
Anticholinergic	Low	Low	Mild	Low	High
Weight gain	Mild	Rare	High	Moderate	High
Type 2 diabetes	Rare	Mild	Moderate	Mild	Moderate
Dyslipidaemia	Rare	Rare	High	Mild	High
Sedation	Low	Mild	Moderate	Mild	High
Sexual dysfunction	Moderate	Mild	Mild	Moderate	Mild
Prolonged QTc interval	High	Mild	Mild	Mild	High
Raised prolactin	High	Rare	Mild	High	Rare

• Sleep disturbances including insomnia and vivid dreams

e) Side Effects of Antipsychotics[6]

It is important to consider the side effect profile of drugs before prescribing for a patient, as in Figure 12.1. For example, if a patient is underweight, an antipsychotic which is associated with weight gain may be preferable, and for a patient who is finding it difficult to sleep, a sedative antipsychotic prescribed at night might be preferable.

Table 12.2 demonstrates the properties of a selection of antipsychotic medications as an indication of the variety of side effects each antipsychotic can have.

Management of these side effects will need to be approached with care and tailored to the patient, and if severe, the choice of antipsychotic medication may need to be changed to one with a more preferable side effect profile.

Text Box 12.3

EPSEs Associated With Antipsychotics

Pseudoparkinsonism: reversible side effects including hand *tremors*, *rigidity* and *bradykinesia*.

Akathisia: a subjective feeling of *inner restlessness* which a patient often feels unable to overcome.

Acute dystonia: increased *spasmic muscle contraction*, which can include an *oculogyric crisis*, *torticollis* and *trismus*.

Tardive dyskinesia: involuntary and *unpredictable body movements*, which commonly effect the face and upper body and can include lip smacking and unusual arm movements. It is associated with long-term antipsychotic use and can be difficult to reverse.

---

f) Metabolic Side Effects of Antipsychotics

Patients who experience *metabolic side effects* are advised to receive specific monitoring and should optimise lifestyle factors as much as possible including[7]:

- Regular exercise.
- A low carbohydrate diet avoiding fast release sugars and high fat foods.
- Body weight monitoring, including weekly for the first six weeks of treatment and then at three months up to one year of treatment. Following this, body weight should be monitored at least once per year or more often if there is rapid weight gain.
- Treatment of any diabetic complications with regular monitoring of Hba1c including three months after starting treatment and then every year.
- Treatment of any dyslipidaemia with statins and regular monitoring of lipid profile initially three months after starting treatment and then yearly.

g) Antipsychotic Associated Hyperprolactinaemia[8]

All antipsychotic medications can lead to raised prolactin levels due to the *blockade of dopamine*, which usually *inhibits prolactin* release. This can be asymptomatic or associated with side effects including gynecomastia, galactorrhoea, sexual dysfunction, reversible infertility and osteoporosis. It is advised that, on admission and prior to any changes or initiation in antipsychotic medication, a baseline prolactin level should be taken.

Clomipramine, *haloperidol*, *amisulpride* and *risperidone* are antipsychotics which are associated with a high risk of hyperprolactinaemia.

Clozapine, olanzapine and *aripiprazole* are antipsychotics associated with a low risk of hyperprolactinaemia.

If a patient's prolactin level is significantly raised and especially if they are symptomatic, this should be fully investigated as per local trust guidelines. But, if it is felt to be due to the antipsychotic, then there are a number of treatment options available. These can be remembered with the mnemonic DASH:

- **D**ose reduction
- **A**djunct therapy with aripiprazole or rarely with dopamine agonists, for example, bromocriptine (can minimise beneficial effect of antipsychotic)
- **S**witching to an alternative antipsychotic
- **H**ormonal therapy led by a specialist

h) Drug Doses

Table 12.3 Doses of antipsychotics (1) (4)

Antipsychotic	Range of daily oral dosing
Chlorpromazine	75–300 mg
Haloperidol	2–10 mg
Sulpiride	200–800 mg
Amisulpride	400–1200 mg
Aripiprazole	10–15 mg
Olanzapine	5–20 mg
Quetiapine	300–750 mg
Risperidone	2–10 mg

Table 12.5 Doses of benzodiazepines (see endnote 2)[9,10]

Benzodiazepine	Approximate dose equivalent to 10 mg diazepam	Half life (hours)
Diazepam	10 mg	20–80 hrs
Clonazepam	1–2 mg	18–50 hrs
Lorazepam	1 mg	10–20 hrs
Chlordiazepoxide	25 mg	5–30 hrs
Temazepam	20 mg	8–15 hrs
Oxazepam	30 mg	5–15 hrs

i) Neuroleptic Malignant Syndrome and Serotonin Syndrome[11]

Neuroleptic malignant syndrome (NMS) and serotonin syndrome are two overlapping conditions caused by treatment with psychotropic medication. They occur rarely but can be life threatening and therefore it is important that they are recognised early on in their presentation and treated as swiftly as possible with cessation of the responsible agent and admission to a physical health hospital with supportive and active treatment as is necessary; these patients often require admission to an intensive care facility. Table 12.6 demonstrates some of the key similarities and differences between the two presentations.

Table 12.6 NMS vs. serotonin syndrome

Neuroleptic malignant syndrome (NMS)	Serotonin syndrome
Precipitated by *dopaminergic agents* such as haloperidol, clozapine and promethazine	Precipitated by *serotonergic agents* such as SSRIs, TCAs, SNRIs, amphetamines, tramadol, ondansetron, St. John's wort.
Gradual onset that might be unpredictable	*Abrupt* onset (usually less than 24 hours), often triggered by combining serotonin enhancing drugs.
Prolonged recovery	*Resolves rapidly.*
Hypertension, tachycardia, hyperthermia	
Rigidity	*Myoclonus* and *tremor.*
Reduced reflexes	*Increased* reflexes.
Normal pupils	*Dilated* pupils.
Treatment involves: Stopping the responsible agent and supportive treatment. Intubation and intensive care support may be required in acute presentations. Benzodiazepines are often used in treatment.	
Bromocriptine, amantadine or dantrolene may be used by specialists.	Treatment with bromocriptine, dantrolene or propranolol is NOT recommended.
Electroconvulsive therapy (ECT) may be required in severe treatment resistant NMS.	

j) Allergies and Toxicity

Table 12.7 Allergies and Toxicity

Blood dyscrasias	Psychotropic medications such as *clozapine, carbamazepine* and *sodium valproate* can lead to blood dyscrasias. Importantly, clozapine is associated with *neutropenia* and *agranulocytosis*, which occur rarely but can potentially be fatal.
Hepatotoxicity	A wide variety of psychotropic medications have been linked with hepatotoxicity including some antidepressants, antipsychotics and mood stabilisers. *Sodium valproate* and *carbamazepine* in particular are associated with hepatotoxicity.
Skin reactions	Many medications used in all fields of medicine can be associated with rashes and allergic reactions. One severe type of reaction associated with *lamotrigine, carbamazepine* and *sertraline,* amongst other medications, is *Stevens-Johnson syndrome* (SJS). This is a severe adverse skin reaction to certain medications that affects the mucous membranes and requires immediate specialist treatment, often in an intensive care unit.[12] Toxic epidermal necrolysis is thought to be part of the same spectrum of severe adverse skin reactions related to medications as SJS.

(Continued)

Table 12.7 (Continued)

Myocarditis	*Myocarditis* is associated with *clozapine* use and should always be considered in a patient presenting with chest pain on clozapine.
Cardiomyopathy	Drug induced cardiomyopathy from psychiatric medications is specifically associated with *clozapine* and *phenothiazines* as well as other medications used outside of psychiatric settings such as chemotherapy drugs and antiretrovirals.[13]
Prolonged QTc and Torsade's de Points	Antipsychotics and antidepressants are associated with prolonged QTc intervals, which can lead to the life threatening arrythmia *Torsade's de Points*. Some antipsychotics such as *haloperidol* and *ziprasidone* are associated with a higher risk of QTc prolongation, whilst *aripiprazole* and *olanzapine* are associated with a lower risk of QTc prolongation.[14],[15] Careful electrocardiogram (ECG) monitoring is required in patients with known cardiac co-morbidities and any patients on antipsychotic medication, especially when high dose antipsychotics are prescribed, requires regular ECG monitoring.

k) Specialist Drug Monitoring

Some medications require specialist drug monitoring either due to their side effect profile or due to having a narrow therapeutic index range where drug efficacy is high, and any side effects or toxicity are minimised.[16]

Two important examples used in psychiatry, *clozapine* and *lithium* are described in more detail in the tables later in this section. Clozapine is an example of a medication that requires careful review due to its side effect profile and lithium is a medication that requires careful monitoring due to its narrow therapeutic index range. Other drugs with a narrow therapeutic index range include carbamazepine, phenytoin, ciclosporin, digoxin and warfarin.

Text Box 12.4

Abbreviations

> Full blood count = FBC
> Liver function tests = LFTs
> Urine and electrolytes = U and Es
> Thyroid function tests = TFTs
> Haemoglobin A1c = HBA1c
> Electrocardiogram = ECG

Clozapine[17,18]

Clozapine is an atypical antipsychotic that is used in *treatment resistant schizo-phrenia*. It can have excellent clinical effects but is only used once at least two

Table 12.8 Clozapine prescribing

Before starting	• Physical examination • Blood tests: FBC, LFTs, U and Es, lipid profile and fasting glucose, HbA1c and prolactin • ECG
Initiation	Monitoring is by a licenced patient monitoring service. Registration is required with the specific brand being used. Starting dose is usually 12.5 mg a day. This is increased slowly over a few weeks and titrated to response and side effects.
Monitoring	• FBC once a week for the first 18 weeks • Then every other week until one year • Every four weeks after one year • Review long-term treatment every three to six months
Forgotten dose	If a single dose is forgotten this should be taken as soon as possible. If more than one clozapine dose has been forgotten, the patient needs to inform the prescriber as re-titration may be required.
Side effects	Common: • Drowsiness • Constipation • Hypersalivation • Tachycardia • Weight gain and raised blood glucose Rarer and more serious: • Reduced white blood cell count (neutropenia) is seen in three in 100 patients. A more severe and life threatening low white blood cell count, agranulocytosis, is seen in one in 100 patients • Myocarditis • Seizures—seizure threshold is lowered
Interactions	Any drugs that inhibit CYP450 isoenzymes may affect plasma levels of clozapine. The main isoenzymes involved in clozapine metabolism are *CYP3A4* and *CYP2D6*. *Cigarette smoking* increases clozapine metabolism and therefore changes in smoking habit often require clozapine dose adjustments. *Caffeine* can lead to increased plasma levels of clozapine. *SSRIs* affect clozapine metabolism via inhibition of CYP2D6. *Antibiotics* such as erythromycin and ciprofloxacin can increase clozapine levels. Clozapine can lead to an *increased chance of NMS* when used with other drugs, such as lithium, which are known to precipitate NMS.

other antipsychotic medications have been tried without adequate therapeutic effect. Clozapine requires close monitoring and has a number of serious side effects and therefore careful consideration is required prior to prescribing the medication.

Lithium[19]

Lithium is a mood stabiliser used in the treatment of bipolar affective disorder. It has a *narrow therapeutic index* and therefore careful monitoring is required as outside this safe range, serious side effects and potentially lethal toxicity can occur, as per Table 12.9.

Table 12.9 Lithium prescribing

Before starting	• Physical examination • Blood tests: FBC, LFTs, U and Es, TFTs • ECG
Initiation	Lithium is prescribed by brand and the dosing will vary according to the brand and the clinical presentation. Lithium trough levels should be checked 12 hours after the last dose, one week after starting the medication.
Monitoring	Once stable, lithium levels can be checked every three to six months. TFTs and an ECG should be performed every six months. Therapeutic range 0.4–1.2 mmol/L (up to 1mmol/l is suitable for most patients).
Forgotten dose	If a single dose is forgotten this should be taken as soon as possible. If more than one lithium dose has been forgotten, the patient needs to inform the prescriber.
Side effects	Common: • Polydipsia • Polyuria (can precipitate nephrogenic diabetes insipidus) • Metallic taste • Fine tremor (course tremor is seen in lithium toxicity) Long-term: • Weight gain • Kidney damage • SIADH • Hypothyroidism • ECG changes (T wave flattening) • Skin changes for example acne and can worsen psoriasis Rarer: • Drowsiness • Double vision • Oedema • Sexual dysfunction Acute toxicity: • **C**ourse tremor • **A**taxia • **N**ausea and vomiting • **C**oma and confusion • **A**cute renal failure • **N**ystagmus This can be recalled by the mnemonic CANCAN.
Interactions	Diuretics, non-steroidal anti-inflammatory drugs, haloperidol, angiotensin-converting enzyme (ACE) inhibitors, SSRIs, carbamazepine. Those prescribed lithium should be advised not to drink alcohol, as it can lead to increased drowsiness and sedation.

l) Prescribing in Special Groups

Children and adolescents	Caution is needed and specialist advice should be sought from a child and adolescent psychiatrist with guidance from a medication formulary for children. *Lower doses* and *different medication protocols* are indicated.

Low weight, elderly and those with intellectual disability	Caution with medication doses is required in specialist groups such as in low weight patients, the elderly and those with learning disabilities, as lower doses may have more profound effects. Consider consulting a pharmacist and starting with *lower doses* and *increasing in smaller increments*.
	It is important to consider significant physiological and pharmacokinetic changes that occur in specialist patient groups. For example, there is a *decrease in plasma protein binding capacity* due to lower albumin levels in the elderly as well as a *reduced renal filtration* rate and *changes in hepatic function*. In anorexic patients, pharmacokinetics can change due to *reduced muscle mass*, wasting and cachexia, *electrolyte disturbance* and significant *reduction in body fat*.
Obesity	*Larger medication doses* may be required, especially for drugs that are lipid soluble drugs due to an *increased volume of distribution*. Consider consulting a pharmacist, as doses above recommended levels may need to be considered. Intramuscular injections might also be troublesome if adipose tissue prevents the injection reaching the muscle below. Adaptations such as *longer needles* may be required.
Co-morbidities	Special consideration is needed in patients with co-morbidities, including renal failure, heart failure and liver failure.
	Examples include:
	• **Liver failure:** using *oxazepam* is preferable to chlordiazepoxide for alcohol withdrawal.[20] Oxazepam is only metabolised by hepatic phase 2 metabolism, which is less affected in liver disease, whereas chlordiazepoxide relies on phase 1 metabolism, which is affected in liver disease.
	• **Kidney failure:** avoid using *lithium* as a mood stabiliser and consider *sodium valproate* instead.
Pregnancy and breastfeeding	Special considerations are required due to the physiological, pharmacokinetic and pharmacodynamic changes that occur and affect many medications during pregnancy. There are significant changes in most body systems including the cardiovascular, renal, respiratory, endocrine and haematological systems.
	An example includes volume changes in the mother leading to *higher doses* of medication sometimes being required, especially in the third trimester of pregnancy.
	An awareness of the *safety of the medication for the foetus* and its propensity to *cross the placenta* and *into breast milk* is also required.

m) Prescribing in Pregnancy and Breastfeeding

When prescribing in pregnancy and breastfeeding, it is important to consider the specific risks and benefits for a patient and the unborn or breastfeeding child. Many medications cross freely across the placenta to the foetus or into the breastmilk with varying clinical effects.

Consider the extent of previous or current mental illness, precipitants of relapse and adjustments made to medications in previous pregnancies as well as the support network available to the patient. Think about referral to specialist teams such as the perinatal psychiatry team.

General principles include:

- Involving the patient in decisions.
- Considering swapping to a preferable medication.
- Using the lowest effective dose.
- Considering splitting doses to reduce peak plasma concentrations.
- Considering more regular foetal screening.
- Offering counselling and more frequent outpatient contact.
- Multi-disciplinary team discussion and specialist referral where necessary.

Key teratogenic medications are outlined in Table 12.10.

With teratogenic medications such as lithium and sodium valproate, it is crucial to ensure that *all decisions are clearly documented* and that essential paperwork, for example, risk acknowledgement forms for the Pregnancy Prevention Programme for Sodium Valproate are completed and stored appropriately.

Table 12.10 Teratogenic medications

Lithium	Maximum risk in the first trimester. Increased risk of cardiac malformations including *Ebstein anomaly*[21] although more recently this has been disputed.[22]
Sodium valproate	Seven times increased chance of malformation.[23] Common malformations include *spina bifida, cleft lip/palate, hypospadias, atrial septal defects* and *polydactyly.*

Preferred treatment options for pregnancy are outlined in Table 12.11.

Table 12.11 Prescribing in pregnancy

Antipsychotics	Olanzapine, chlorpromazine, haloperidol, clozapine
Antidepressants	Fluoxetine
Mood stabilisers	No mood stabiliser is recommended; consider antipsychotics
Sedatives	Promethazine, benzodiazepines (to avoid in late pregnancy as can lead to hypotonia and neonatal withdrawal)

Preferred treatment options for breastfeeding are outlined in Table 12.12:

Table 12.12 Prescribing in breastfeeding

Antipsychotics	Olanzapine
Antidepressants	Sertraline

| Mood stabilisers | Avoid, if possible. Sodium valproate is preferred if essential but can lead to hepatotoxicity in the infant and adequate protection against further pregnancy is required. |
| Sedatives | Lorazepam |

n) Principles in Psychiatric Emergencies

All emergencies	In all emergencies, in line with national guidelines, staff should ensure their own safety prior to assessing the patient, call for help and assess the patient using approaches taught in basic and intermediate life support courses in which all staff should have training. An ambulance should be called immediately if there are any physical health concerns. Trust guidelines should be followed where available.
Dystonic reaction[24]	An acute dystonic reaction is characterised by involuntary contractions of muscles of the extremities, face, neck, abdomen, pelvis or larynx in either sustained or intermittent patterns that lead to abnormal movements or postures. The aetiology of an acute dystonic reaction is thought to be due to neurotransmitter imbalance in the basal ganglia. A number of medications can be used in the treatment of dystonic reactions, including *benztropine*, diphenhydramine, benzodiazepines and trihexyphenidyl. Clinicians should *stop the responsible medication* and supportive measures in hospital are advised.
Oculogyric crisis[25],[26]	An oculogyric crisis occurs when there is a spasm of the extraocular muscles leading to tonic, usually upward deviation of the eye. Each spasm can last from seconds to several hours. An oculogyric crisis is associated with the use of medications including antidepressants, antipsychotics and anti-emetics (metoclopramide is strongly associated with precipitating this side effect in females). A number of medications can be used in the treatment of an oculogyric crisis including *benztropine*, diphenhydramine, benzodiazepines and trihexyphenidyl. Clinicians should *stop the responsible medication* and seek further medical support as is necessary.
Neuroleptic malignant syndrome and serotonin syndrome	Early recognition is crucial. Treatment involves *stopping the responsible agent* and *transfer to a physical health hospital*. Supportive treatment is the main treatment; however, benzodiazepines may be used. *Intubation and intensive care* support with specialist drugs may be required.
Hanging	If a patient is found hanging, staff should call for help and ensure that a ligature cutter is used to release the ligature with controlled c-spine stabilisation and support of the head and neck. Ward staff should have training in cutting a ligature and should avoid the knot. An individual cannot do this safely without support from colleagues. Further medical assistance should follow in line with life support guidance and in relation to the injuries sustained. Review of airway patency should be repeated due to possible delayed oropharyngeal oedema.

(Continued)

(Continued)

Deliberate self-harm	Management of a deliberate self-harming incident is dependent on the method of self-harm, any object used to cause injury and the degree of injury caused. Where possible, remove the object used to cause injury and treat any acute medical problems. Ensure that smaller injuries are not neglected and consider reviewing leave and other safety plans in place as well as a risk assessment to ensure patient safety such as removing further objects that may be with the patient that could cause harm to themselves or others.
Medication overdose	If a patient has taken a medication overdose, it is important to ensure they no longer have access to the medication source or stockpile. Depending on the medication or combination of medications that have been taken, a physical health review in the accident and emergency department will be required and, if in doubt, further discussion with an acute hospital physician is suggested. Certain medications will have specific management treatments, for example, *N-acetylcysteine* (NAC) in paracetamol overdose, and specialist advice should be sought with toxicology resources such as TOXBASE referred to for guidance. Certain medications are particularly dangerous in overdose, for example, the TCAs amitriptyline, dosulepin and doxepin and in patients who are high risk of overdose, these should be avoided.
Violent incidents	All violent incidents should be managed in three stages: Acutely, any physical injuries should be attended to, safety prioritised and de-escalation used where possible with physical restraint, rapid tranquilisation and seclusion used as a last resort. The incident should be documented and a safety incident form submitted using the online adverse incident reporting system. A safety huddle or space for reflection should be used within the team to learn from the event.

o) Driving

An in depth understanding of each psychiatric condition and whether the Driver and Vehicle Licensing Agency (DVLA) needs to be informed is not required, however, an understanding of the key principles is important, and these principles are outlined in Table 12.13.[27]

Table 12.13 DVLA advice

Mild to moderate anxiety and depression	*May drive* and the DVLA does not need to be notified as long as there are no significant deficits in cognition, concertation, agitation or suicidal thoughts.
Severe anxiety and depression	*Must not drive* and must *notify the DVLA.*
Acute psychotic disorder	*Must not drive during acute illness* and must *notify the DVLA.*
Mania	*Must not drive during the acute illness* and must *notify the DVLA*, but *can drive after a manic episode* if certain conditions are met.

Schizophrenia	*Must not drive during the acute illness* and must *notify the DVLA*, but *can drive after a manic episode* if certain conditions are met.
Mild cognitive impairment	*May drive* and the DVLA does not need to be notified.
Dementia	*Must notify the DVLA.* There is acknowledgement that dementia can present in different ways with alternative rates of progression and the decision on licensing is usually based on medical reports with review as is necessary.
Mild learning disability	*Must notify the DVLA.* Licensing will be granted providing there are no other significant relevant problems.
Severe learning disability	*Must NOT drive* and must *notify the DVLA.*

p) Electroconvulsive Therapy (ECT)

Electroconvulsive therapy (ECT) is a treatment that has been successfully used in the treatment of psychiatric disorders since the 1930s. It involves using one or two electrodes that are placed on a patient's scalp to induce a seizure. The patient is under an anaesthetic during the procedure and is given a muscle relaxant. It is not painful, and the main associated difficulties related to ECT are the *anaesthetic and the anaesthetic recovery* as well as transient *fatigue, confusion, nausea, headache* and in some cases *short-term memory loss*.

ECT is used in the management of depression, acute mania, catatonia and treatment resistant schizophrenia. The therapeutic response achieved through ECT is usually more rapid than using psychotropic medications and can be lifesaving in many cases including acute catatonic states where a patient is not eating or drinking.

The exact mechanism behind the therapeutic effect of ECT is not clear, but there are three main categories of hypothesis: neurophysiological, neurobiochemical and neuroplasticity theories.[28]

- **Neurophysiological hypothesis**: The electrical impulse from the ECT electrodes stimulates neurons and alters concentrations of ions in the brain, leading to a seizure. This could lead to changes in cerebral blood flow and regional metabolism, changes in the blood brain barrier and other changes in the higher functionality of the brain, which can be seen in electroencephalographic changes.
- **Neurobiochemical hypothesis**: ECT affects neurotransmission and influences the expression and release of neurochemicals in brain. These changes include changes in transcription factors, neurotransmitters, neurotrophic factors and hormones.
- **Neuroplasticity hypothesis**: Studies have shown that ECT can lead to visible changes in the appearance of the brain, as can be seen in neuroimaging. This includes changes in volume of whole brain as well as changes in grey matter, white matter and specific brain structures, suggesting changes in neuronal connections on a large scale.

q) Factors Affecting Medication Adherence[29]

Table 12.14 Factors affecting medication adherence

Demographic	• Sex
	• Gender
	• Ethnicity
Psycho-social	• Religious and cultural beliefs
	• Educational background
	• Alcohol, tobacco and recreational drug use
Personal	• Understanding of the treatment and reasons for use
	• Perceived risk/benefit
	• Co-morbidities including mental health and insight
	• Relationship status
	• Previous medication use and compliance
Treatment related	• Route of administration
	• Duration of treatment
	• Side effects of medication
	• Number of doses
	• Timing of doses
Practical	• Ease of access to prescription
	• Transport availability
	• Physical mobility

r) The Placebo Effect

The placebo effect is a psychological phenomenon that refers to a medication or intervention that does not have an effect with therapeutic value but results in an outcome that cannot be attributed to the placebo's intrinsic properties.

This can lead to significantly different outcomes in individuals' experiences of taking a medication and as a result, clinical trials often have a control arm to mitigate the placebo effect from affecting the results.

Notes

1. British National Formulary. [Online] https://bnf.nice.org.uk.
2. Dean, Laura. (2015). Carbamazepine Therapy and HLA Genotype. Medical Genetics Summaries. gov.uk.
3. British National Formulary. [Online] https://bnf.nice.org.uk.
4. [Online] www.mind.org.uk/information-support/drugs-and-treatments/antidepressants/side-effects-of-antidepressants/.
5. Sweet, R. A., E. J. Brown, R. G. Heimberg, L. Ciafre, D. M. Scanga, J. R. Cornelius, S. Dube, K. M. Forsyth, and C. S. Holt. (1995). Monoamine Oxidase Inhibitor Dietary Restrictions: What Are We Asking Patients to Give Up? *Journal of Clinical Psychiatry*, 56 (5).
6. Hamer, J. M., and M. Ann. (2010). Adverse Effects of Antipsychotic Medications. *American Family Physician*, 81 (5).
7. [Online] https://cks.nice.org.uk/topics/psychosis-schizophrenia/prescribing-information/monitoring/.
8. Moustafa, Hany F., B. Rizk, A. Helvacioglu, and S. Gilmore. (2018). *Hyperprolactinaemia: A Guide for Psychiatrists*. Cambridge: Cambridge University Press.

9. Taylor, P. K. (2015). *The Maudsley Prescribing Guidelines in Psychiatry.* New York. Wiley Blackwell; British National Formulary.

10. Charles E. Griffin, III, A. M. Kaye, F. Rivera Bueno, and A. D. Kaye. (2013). Benzodiazepine Pharmacology and Central Nervous System – Mediated Effects. *The Ochner Journal,* 13.

11. Kateon, H. (2013). Differentiating Serotonin Syndrome and Neuroleptic Malignant Syndrome. *Mental Health Clinician,* 3.

12. [Online] www.nhs.uk/conditions/stevens-johnson-syndrome/.

13. Albakri, A. (2019). Drugs-Related Cardiomyopathy: A Systematic Review and Pooled Analysis of Pathophysiology, Diagnosis and Clinical Management. *Internal Medicine and Care,* 3.

14. Hamer, J. M., and M. Ann. (2010). Adverse Effects of Antipsychotic Medications. *American Family Physician,* 81 (5).

15. Dietle, Aimee. (2015). QTc Prolongation with Antidepressants and Antipsychotics. *US Pharm,* 40 (11).

16. Blix, Hege S., Kirsten K. Viktil, Tron A. Moger, and A. Reikvam. (2010). Drugs with Narrow Therapeutic Index as Indicators in the Risk Management of Hospitalised Patients. *Pharmacology Practice,* 8 (1).

17. www.sussexpartnership.nhs.uk/sites/default/files/documents/clozapine_guidance_-_combined_-_dec_15_-_other_medicines_warning_added.pdf.

18. [Online] www.slam.nhs.uk/media/19073/clozapine.pdf.

19. [Online] https://slam.nhs.uk/media/18276/lithium.pdf.

20. Peppers, M. (1996). Benzodiazepines for Alcohol Withdrawal in the Elderly and Patients with Liver Disease. *Pharmacotherapy,* 16.

21. Poels, Eline M. P., Hilmar H. Bijma, Megan Galbally, and Veerle Bergink. (2018). Lithium During Pregnancy and After Delivery: A Review. *International Journal of Bipolar Disorders,* 6 (26).

22. [Online] www.rcpsych.ac.uk/mental-health/treatments-and-wellbeing/lithium-in-pregnancy-and-breastfeeding.

23. Macfarlane, Alastair, and Trisha Greenhalgh. (2018). Sodium Valproate in Pregnancy: What Are the Risks and Should We Use a Shared Decision-Making Approach? *BMC Pregnancy Childbirth,* 18 (200).

24. Lewis, K., and C. S. O'Day. (2021). Dystonic Reactions. In *StatPearls* [Internet]. Treasure Island, FL: StatPearls Publishing.

25. Kaski, D., and A. M. Bronstein. (2016). Functional Eye Movement Disorders. *Handbook of Clinical Neurology.* Amsterdam: Elsevier; Liu, G. T., N. J. Volpe, and S. Galetta. (2010). *Eye Movement Disorders. Neuro-Ophthalmology: Diagnosis and Management.* Philadelphia: Saunders Elsevier, 2nd ed., pp. 491–550.

26. Liu, G. T., Volpe, N. J., and Galetta, S. L. (2010). *Eye Movement Disorders. Neuro-Ophthalmology: Diagnosis and Management.* Philadelphia, PA: Saunders Elsevier, 2nd ed., pp. 491–550.

27. [Online] www.gov.uk/guidance/psychiatric-disorders-assessing-fitness-to-drive.

28. Kar, Amit Singh, and Sujita Kumar. (2017). How Electroconvulsive Therapy Works? Understanding the Neurobiological Mechanisms. *Clinical Psychopharmacology Neuroscience,* 15.

29. Jin, Jing, Grant Edward Sklar, Vernon Min Sen Oh, and Shu Chuen Li. (2008). Factors Affecting Therapeutic Compliance: A Review from the Patient's Perspective. *Therapeutic Clinical Risk Management,* 4.

13 Pharmacokinetics

Lisanne Stock

a) Key Aspects

It is important to understand the difference between pharmacodynamics and pharmacokinetics.

Pharmacodynamics describes the effect of a *drug on the body* and is determined by complex chemical interactions reliant on cascades on a cellular level and *interactions between a medication and the binding site* at a receptor, for example, the mechanisms of action of psychotropic drugs.

Pharmacokinetics refers to the effect of the *body on the drug*, which is related to the *time course* and *disposition* of the drug once in the body.

A drug may be given by varying *routes of administration*, which may influence the pharmacokinetics of that same drug. Psychotropic medications are most commonly given via oral, parenteral (intramuscular and intravenous) or transcutaneous (rectal and sublingual) routes to enter the systemic system to reach the target organ (the brain). This movement around the body may occur *independently* of drug chemistry via *bulk flow*, or *dependent* on the drug chemistry across cell barriers via *diffusion* and *active transport*.

Molecules that are *lipid-soluble* will *diffuse* across cell membranes moving from a region of higher to lower concentration, *down the concentration gradient*. This is because cell membranes are made of lipoproteins.

Molecules that are *non-lipid-soluble* will be *transported* across cell membranes via *carrier mechanisms* or *aqueous channels*.

The *bioavailability* of a drug is the proportion that reaches its target to have an active effect. It is concerned with four key principles: *M*etabolism, *A*bsorption, *D*istribution and *E*xcretion (*MADE*).[1]

b) Absorption

Absorption is the movement of a drug into the bloodstream after administration. The rate of absorption is influenced by:

- *Solubility*—gastric and intestinal pH affect solubility, as does pKa (the acid dissociation constant, the pH at which half of the drug will be in its

DOI: 10.1201/9781003322573-18

ionised form). Hydrophobic drugs quickly permeate the lipid cell membranes lining the gut and are therefore more quickly absorbed than hydrophilic drugs. For this reason, only 40% of a chlorpromazine dose will reach the systemic circulation.

- *Blood flow* at the site of drug administration.
- Drug *delivery systems*, such as long acting injectable (LAI) drugs or enteric coated drugs.

Oral preparations are most commonly used in psychiatry, but the absorption is often erratic, leading to variable plasma concentrations. Drugs are also subject to 'first-pass metabolism' in the liver, occurring before entering the systemic circulation. If the liver is damaged, hepatic impairment might reduce first-pass metabolism, requiring the dosages to be adjusted.

Oral preparations must be soluble in stomach acid and, resistant to the acid pH and be lipid soluble to allow for passive diffusion across cell membranes.

Erratic absorption is influenced by various factors such as gastric pH, intestinal microbiomes, surface area of gastrointestinal tract available, blood flow, presence of food and gastric motility.

Text Box 13.1

P-glycoprotein reverse transporter pumps actively remove some drugs, by an adenosine triphosphate dependent process, depositing them back into the gut lumen and reducing the absorption rate.

Grapefruit juice is a potent inhibitor of P-glycoprotein, which increases drug oral bioavailability. This effect is greatest for drugs with high first-pass metabolism such as carbamazepine, midazolam and simvastatin.

Parenteral administration includes intravenous (IV) and intramuscular (IM) injection. IV absorption occurs most quickly, with IM occurring over 10–30 minutes. IV administration leads to 100% bioavailability as there is no 'first-pass' metabolism. Both routes avoid first-pass metabolism. LAIs have deliberately slowed absorption by use of inert oils, salts and encapsulation techniques.

c) Distribution

Distribution of a drug refers to its movement within the body after absorption from the gut. This continues until equilibrium of the drug throughout body compartments has occurred.

The two-compartment system models a drug moving from the central compartment, plasma, into peripheral compartments, such as the brain, fat and bones. As distribution occurs, the plasma concentration will inevitably be lower.

Distribution is related to various factors including plasma protein binding, tissue perfusion, tissue membrane permeability and active transport out of tissues.

Text Box 13.2

Plasma protein binding can significantly alter the availability and distribution of drugs within the body. If plasma protein binding is high, there is a large reservoir of the drug available in the intravascular compartment for delivery to the effect site.

If a patient has large physiological disruptions, for example, albumin changes in patients with liver disease, or if they are post-surgery or pregnancy, it can have a significant effect on protein binding and the distribution of drugs. It is for this reason that certain patient groups often require medication adjustments, including dosage and choice of medication. Certain medications can affect the protein binding of others, such as sodium (Na) valproate, which is able to displace other medications such as phenytoin from protein binding sites.

Text Box 13.3

Volume of distribution $(V_d) = Q/C_p$
  Q = quantity of drug; C_p = plasma concentration
  The higher the V_d, the lower the plasma concentration
  The lower the V_d, the higher the plasma concentration
  A high V_d suggests the drug has affinity for tissues in the peripheral compartments such as the brain and fat in tissue compartments rather than the circulating plasma.

When in the blood, a fraction of most drugs will be protein bound, leaving the unbound fraction to be active. The fraction of a drug that is protein bound is usually in equilibrium, but when altered can lead to an increase in the unbound, active fraction. When renal disease is present leading to proteinuria, this phenomenon must be considered. The relevance is most profound for drugs that are highly protein bound, such as phenytoin. Diazepam in recognised as a common cause of phenytoin displacement from its protein bindings, leading to a potential increase in side effects. In most other examples of this, the effect is limited because metabolism of the drug will increase to compensate.

Drugs that are highly protein bound tend to accumulate in high plasma concentrations, as that is where the protein exists, leading to a lowed V_d.

The **blood-brain barrier** (BBB) has an important role in the distribution and availability of drugs in the central nervous system.[2] It influences the passage of substances from the blood plasma via *tight junctions* between the capillary endothelial cells. Only lipid-soluble molecules can enter the brain via this route, otherwise passive transport (lithium ions) or active transport (L-dopa, L-tryptophan and valproate) is required.

The integrity of the BBB can be more permeable when inflamed.

Circumventricular regions such as the *median eminence of the hypothalamus* and the *vomiting centre* are areas of the brain not protected by the BBB. Nasal sprays can also bypass the BBB to some extent.

d) Metabolism

Metabolism is the conversion of a drug into a *more water-soluble* and less lipid-soluble form, to allow for its elimination from the body. This primarily takes places in the liver but can occur at other sites including the gastrointestinal tract, blood plasma, kidneys and lungs, among other areas. Metabolism is usually the rate limiting step in pharmacokinetics, apart from for lithium, which being a salt, is eliminated unaltered.

Phase 1 metabolism: is usually mediated via *cytochrome P450* (CYP) enzymes[3] and sometimes via *flavin containing mono-oxygenase* (FMO). This occurs through the processes of *oxidation, reduction* and *hydrolysis*, but most psychotropic drugs undergo oxidation via CYP.

After phase 1 metabolism, the product may be more or less active than the parent compound. Not all drugs undergo phase 1 metabolism, for example lorazepam, oxazepam and temazepam (**LOT**), which therefore have preferred use for alcohol detoxification where liver disease is significant.

Text Box 13.4

Medications which undergo little hepatic metabolism include:

Lithium
Amisulpride
Sulpiride
Acamprosate
Amantadine
Gabapentin

These, therefore, mostly undergo renal elimination.

Text Box 13.5

Cytochrome P450 enzymes

CYP2D6 and CYP3A4 are responsible for the metabolism of 90% of psychotropic medications, where they act in the endoplasmic reticulum of hepatocytes and cells of the intestine.

Genetic variations in hepatic enzymes exist:

The CYP2D6 isoenzyme is lacking in 5–10% of Caucasians and 1–2% of Asians, leading to poor metabolism of its substrates (aripiprazole, citalopram, risperidone and tricyclics).

The CYP2C19 isoenzyme is lacking in 20% of East Asians, leading to poor metabolism of diazepam and citalopram.

Text Box 13.6

Inducers increase CYP450 enzyme activity by increasing enzyme synthesis. This can lead to a decrease in plasma concentration of drugs metabolised by the CYP450 system.

Inducers:

Carbamazepine
Barbiturates
Tobacco
St John's wort
Phenytoin
Rifampicin

Can be remembered by the nmemonic CBT SPR.

Inhibitors reduce CYP450 enzyme activity by reducing enzyme synthesis. This can lead to an increase in plasma concentration of drugs metabolised by the CYP450 system.

Inhibitors:

Antidepressants: specifically, fluoxetine and paroxetine
Antibiotics: specifically, ciprofloxacin, isoniazid and metronidazole
Antifungal: specifically, fluconazole
Anti-retroviral: specifically, ritonavir and indinavir

Metabolism of sertraline is via multiple pathways, meaning that reduced activity of an individual CYP isoenzyme will be less influential to its overall metabolism.

Some psychotropics drugs, whilst being metabolised by CYP, can also inhibit or induce CYP metabolism, which has the following clinical relevance:

Fluvoxamine can inhibit clozapine metabolism at CYP1A2, leading to a 10x increase in plasma levels.

Fluoxetine can inhibit tricyclic antidepressant (TCA) metabolism at CYP2D6 and CYP 2C19.

Carbamazepine can induce CYP activity, leading to increased metabolism and decreased plasma concentration of oral contraception.

Alcohol and smoking are CYP inducers, with smoking leading to a significant reduction in clozapine plasma levels. Smoking also affects olanzapine plasma levels, to some degree.

Grapefruit juice and caffeine are inhibitors of the CYP system.

Phase 2 metabolism usually involves the phase 1 metabolites undergoing *conjugation* with glucuronic acid (*glucuronidation*). This produces polar (water-soluble) compounds which are excretable in the bile or in the urine. If the relative molecular mass is less than 300, the compound is excreted via the kidneys, and if over 300, excretion is in the bile.

Valproate can reduce the glucuronidation of lamotrigine, leading to increased plasma concentrations.

Drugs competing for the same metabolic pathway, such as TCAs and haloperidol, will decreased the metabolism of both.

Liver impairment, from direct injury or old age, will decrease the metabolism of most psychotropic drugs.

Most antidepressants are known to *inhibit warfarin metabolism*, leading to an increased risk of serious bleeding.

Some drugs induce their own metabolism (*auto-induction*), such as carbamazepine and phenobarbitone. Therefore, the rate of metabolism gradually increases over the first weeks of treatment, meaning steady state will be delayed.

Amitriptyline and clomipramine can increase the risk of opioid toxicity, as they will inhibit the metabolism of morphine.

Text Box 13.7

Antidepressants with active metabolites:

Fluoxetine	→	Norfluoxetine
Sertraline	→	Desmethylsertraline
Amitriptyline	→	Nortriptyline
Imipramine	→	Desipramine

e) Excretion[4,5]

Excretion of drugs is usually via *urine*, faeces or in bile. It should also be noted that excretion of both active and inactive metabolites can also occur in breast milk and sweat.

Non-lipid soluble and *ionised* compounds are most suited to excretion via the kidneys, lithium being a good example of this.

Excretion is affected by:

- Increased age, leading to decreased excretion
- Decreased renal blood flow, for example, as a result of dehydration, decreased glomerular filtration rate (GFR), or medications such as non-steroidal anti-inflammatory drugs (NSAIDs)
- Altered reabsorption due to changes in urine pH. Low Na causes increases in lithium reabsorption and therefore decreased excretion

---

Text Box 13.8

Clearance (Cl) = rate of elimination (metabolism + excretion) of a
           drug
           = volume of blood cleared by the drug, per unit of time
Clearance is directly proportional to Vd such that
      $Cl = k \times Vd$
      k = 'the first order elimination constant'

The *half-life* ($t_{1/2}$) (Figure 13.1) is the time taken for the plasma concentration to fall by 50%.

Distribution half-life refers specifically to the time taken for a plasma concentration to fall by 50% due to redistribution from the plasma into body tissues after IV administration.

Elimination half-life refers specifically to the time taken for a plasma concentration to fall by 50% due to metabolism and excretion.

Drugs with longer $T_{1/2}$, which is close to 24 hours, such as tricyclics, will be dosed once daily.

Steady state refers to a defined degree of consistency in plasma concentrations despite frequent administrations of the drug. It is said to have been achieved when the average plasma concentration between two successive doses remains the same, that is, rate in = rate out. It is independent of the frequency of administration. It usually takes 4.5 half-lives for a drug to reach a 'steady-state' plasma levels, if there is repeated administration of that drug.

If the drug is administered at greater intervals than the $t_{1/2}$, there will be large fluctuations in the plasma concentration.

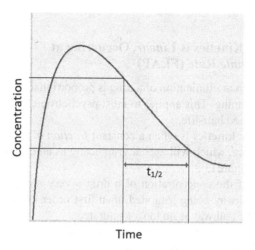

Figure 13.1 Plasma drug concentration curve

Loading doses (large initial doses) can achieve steady state more quickly, for example treating mania with valproate.

Area under the curve (AUC) (Figure 13.1) after a single dose is proportional to the plasma concentration and allows the bioavailability to be calculated from the fraction of the dose that is absorbed.

The *therapeutic index* refers to the difference between the minimum therapeutic concentrations and the minimum toxic concentrations in the blood. Medications with a narrow therapeutic index, such as lithium and phenytoin, require only minor dose adjustments before they become harmful. In the examples, careful monitoring of plasma concentration is necessary.

Text Box 13.9

First-Order Kinetics is *Linear*, Occurring at A *Proportionate* Rate (FLAP)

The absorption or elimination of a drug is proportional to the amount of the drug remaining. This applies to most psychotropic drugs and corresponds to a fixed half-life.

First-order kinetics is when a constant *fraction* of a drug is cleared per unit of time, which will appear graphically as an exponential decay curve, as in Figure 13.2.

However, if the concentration of a drug a very high, leading to its metabolic pathway being saturated, then first order kinetics might not occur until the pathway is no longer saturated.

Zero-order kinetics is when absorption or elimination of a drug is at a constant fixed *amount*, *independent* of the amount of the drug remaining. This is seen with controlled release drugs and LAIs (depots).

Linearity means that if the dose of a drug is increased, the plasma concentration will increase proportionally. This is not valid for some drugs, such as alcohol and phenytoin, which follow *dose-dependent kinetics*.

The significance of linearity is demonstrated with SSRIs. Sertraline and citalopram follow linear pharmacokinetics, the $T_{1/2}$ for a single dose and multiple doses is unchanged. Fluoxetine and paroxetine follow non-linear pharmacokinetics. The $T_{1/2}$ for a single dose of fluoxetine is 1.9 days, whereas after multiple doses, it is 5.6 days. The $T_{1/2}$ for a single dose of paroxetine is ten hours, whereas after multiple doses it is 21 hours. Conversely, the $T_{1/2}$ for citalopram and sertraline is linear and therefore unchanged, irrespective of single or multiple doses.

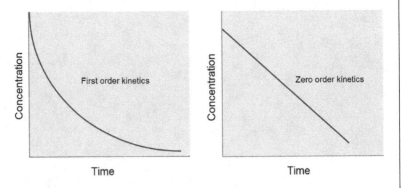

Figure 13.2 First order and zero order kinetics

Factors affecting pharmacokinetics:

Old age is responsible for[6]:

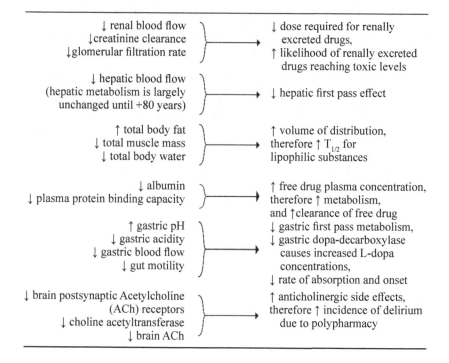

↓ renal blood flow ↓creatinine clearance ↓glomerular filtration rate	↓ dose required for renally excreted drugs, ↑ likelihood of renally excreted drugs reaching toxic levels
↓ hepatic blood flow (hepatic metabolism is largely unchanged until +80 years)	↓ hepatic first pass effect
↑ total body fat ↓ total muscle mass ↓ total body water	↑ volume of distribution, therefore ↑ $T_{1/2}$ for lipophilic substances
↓ albumin ↓ plasma protein binding capacity	↑ free drug plasma concentration, therefore ↑ metabolism, and ↑clearance of free drug
↑ gastric pH ↓ gastric acidity ↓ gastric blood flow ↓ gut motility	↓ gastric first pass metabolism, ↓ gastric dopa-decarboxylase causes increased L-dopa concentrations, ↓ rate of absorption and onset
↓ brain postsynaptic Acetylcholine (ACh) receptors ↓ choline acetyltransferase ↓ brain ACh	↑ anticholinergic side effects, therefore ↑ incidence of delirium due to polypharmacy

Renal impairment:

Drugs such as lithium are nephrotoxic and can damage the liver further.

The half-life of diazepam will remain unchanged in renal disease, but active metabolites may accumulate.

Avoid medications which are extensively renally excreted: lithium, sulpiride and amisulpride.

The excretion of risperidone and active metabolites is reduced in renal failure, meaning oral doses should be adjusted accordingly and depot should not be prescribed until this has occurred.

Pregnancy[7]:

Decreased gastro-intestinal motility and delayed gastric emptying during pregnancy both contribute to delayed drug absorption rates.

The glomerular filtration rate usually increases during pregnancy, meaning renal clearance is increased.

An increase in total body water affects distribution, causing lower peak serum concentrations of drugs after absorption.

Albumin levels and therefore protein binding is reduced, leading to increased available drug in its free form.

Notes

1. Currie, Geoffrey M. (2018). Pharmacology, Part 2: Introduction to Pharmacokinetics. *Journal of Nuclear Medicine Technology*, 46.
2. Daneman, Richard, and Alexandre Prat. 2015. The Blood – Brain Barrier. *Cold Spring Harbour Perspectives in Biology*, 7.
3. Lynch, Tom, and Amy Price. (2007). The Effect of Cytochrome P450 Metabolism on Drug Response, Interactions, and Adverse Effects. *American Family Physician*, 76.
4. Horde, Gaither W., and Gupta Vikas. (2021). *Drug Clearance*. Treasure Island, FL: Stat Pearls Publishing.
5. Borowy, Christopher S., and John V. Ashurst. (2020). *Physiology, Zero and First Order Kinetics*. Treasure Island, FL: Stat Pearls Publishing.
6. Taylor, D., C. Paton, and S. Kapur. (2009). *The Maudsley Prescribing Guidelines*. London: CRC Press, pp. 386–387.
7. Loebstein, R., A. Lalkin, and G. Koren. (1997). Pharmacokinetic Changes During Pregnancy and Their Clinical Relevance. *Clinical Pharmacokinetics*, 33 (5): 328–343.

14 Broader Aspects of Psychopharmacology

Lisanne Stock

a) Clinical Trials

All medicines will go through a number of rigorous tests to ensure that they are safe to be used.[1] A medicine or intervention will be tested often against a control so that any clinically significant differences can be identified. A drug will need to go through the following steps in order for it to be approved by a regulatory body; in the UK, this is the Medicines and Healthcare Products Regulatory Agency (MHRA). There are a number of phases to a clinical trial:

Phase I Trial

- A small group of healthy volunteers will be given the medicine to test the safety of the medication.
- Any side effects will be noted.

Phase II Trial

- A larger sample of people will be used to test the medication.
- This group of people will suffer from the disease that the medication or intervention is intended to treat.

Phase III Trial

- If a medicine or intervention has no significant adverse effects in the earlier two stages, it will be tested on a bigger group of people with the illness.
- The aim of this stage is to see if there is any benefit over existing treatment and also to note if there are any significant side effects that weren't observed in a smaller population.
- This stage is often the longest.

DOI: 10.1201/9781003322573-19

Phase IV Trial

- If a medication has passed all previous stages, this phase will be carried out to continue to monitor the safety and side effect profile of the medication over a prolonged period.
- This stage only applies to medications which have been approved to be used by a regulatory body.

Text Box 14.1

Drug Regulation

In the UK, drugs are licensed based upon their known indications and side effects. Most medications used within clinical medicine will be approved to be used for a certain patient group or condition within a defined dosage. Medications that are used off label may be used for medical conditions that they were not originally indicated for or outside the usual dose range. For example, venlafaxine is an antidepressant medication licenced for use in depression, anxiety and panic disorders but is often prescribed off label in attention-deficit/hyperactivity disorder, obsessive compulsive disorder and post-traumatic stress disorder.

---

b) Adverse Event Reporting

Adverse event reporting will vary depending on the guidelines of the employing trust. However, there is a basic outline that should be followed in clinical practice:

- Ensure the acute safety of patients and staff.
- Alert the lead clinician and lead nursing staff on the ward.
- There is a duty of candour to inform the patient and if necessary, their relatives, as soon as possible after the incident.
- The event should be documented in a contemporaneous manner in the clinical notes with adequate detail about what occurred with clear outing of the date and time as well as members of staff involved.
- A local incident should be raised on the reporting system used by the trust, for example, Datix or Ulysses.
- If the adverse event was linked to an adverse drug reaction it should be reported to the MHRA through the Yellow Card Scheme website (https://yellowcard.mhra.gov.uk). Alternatively, prepaid Yellow Cards for reporting adverse drug reactions can be found in the inside cover of the British National Formulary (BNF).
- Consider discussing with a line manager or supervisor.

Note

1. [Online] www.nhs.uk/conditions/clinical-trials/.

Source Material

Albakri, A. (2019). Drugs-Related Cardiomyopathy: A Systematic Review and Pooled Analysis of Pathophysiology, Diagnosis and Clinical Management. *Internal Medicine and Care*, 3.

Blix, Hege S., Kirsten K. Viktil, Tron A. Moger, and Aasmund Reikvam. (2010). Drugs with Narrow Therapeutic Index as Indicators in the Risk Management of Hospitalised Patients. *Pharmacology Practice*, 8 (1).

Borowy, Christopher S., and John V. Ashurst. (2020). *Physiology, Zero and First Order Kinetics*. Treasure Island, FL: StatPearls Publishing.

British National Formulary. [Online] https://bnf.nice.org.uk.

Charles E. Griffin, III, A. M. Kaye, F. Rivera Bueno, and A. D. Kaye. (2013). Benzodiazepine Pharmacology and Central Nervous System – Mediated Effects. *The Ochner Journal*, 13.

Currie, Geoffrey M. (2018). Pharmacology, Part 2: Introduction to Pharmacokinetics. *Journal of Nuclear Medicine Technology*, 46.

Daneman, Richard, and Alexandre Prat. 2015. The Blood – Brain Barrier. *Cold Spring Harbour Perspectives in Biology*, 7.

Dean, Laura. (2015). *Carbamazepine Therapy and HLA Genotype*. Medical Genetics Summaries.

Dietle, Aimee. (2015). QTc Prolongation with Antidepressants and Antipsychotics. *US Pharm*, 40 (11).

Enevoldson, T P. (2004). Recreational drugs and their neurological consequences. *BMJ Journal of Neurology, Neurosurgery and Psychiatry*, 75 (3).

Hamer, J. M., and M. Ann. (2010). Adverse Effects of Antipsychotic Medications. *American Family Physician*, 81 (5).

Horde, Gaither W., and Gupta Vikas. (2021). *Drug Clearance*. Treasure Island, FL: StatPearls Publishing.

Jin, Jing, Grant Edward Sklar, Vernon Min Sen Oh, and Shu Chuen Li. (2008). Factors Affecting Therapeutic Compliance: A Review from the Patient's Perspective. *Therapeutic Clinical Risk Management*, 4.

Kar, Amit Singh, and Sujita Kumar. (2017). How Electroconvulsive Therapy Works? Understanding the Neurobiological Mechanisms. *Clinical Psychopharmacology Neuroscience*, 15.

Kaski, D., and A. M. Bronstein. (2016). *Functional Neurologic Disorders, Handbook of Clinical Neurology*. Amsterdam: Elsevier.

Kateon, Hayley. (2013). Differentiating serotonin syndrome and neuroleptic malignant syndrome. *Mental Health Clinician*, 3.

Lewis, Kevin, and Carla S. O'Day. (2021). *Dystonic Reactions*. In *StatPearls* [Internet]. Treasure Island, FL: StatPearls Publishing.

Liu, Grant T., and Steven L. Galetta. (2010). *Eye Movement Disorders, Neuro-Ophthalmology*. 2nd ed.

Lynch, Tom, and Amy Price. (2007). The Effect of Cytochrome P450 Metabolism on Drug Response, Interactions, and Adverse Effects. *American Family Physician*, 76.

Macfarlane, Alastair, and Trisha Greenhalgh. (2018). Sodium Valproate in Pregnancy: What Are the Risks and Should We Use a Shared Decision-Making Approach? *BMC Pregnancy Childbirth*, 18 (200).

Moustafa, Hany F., Botros Rizk, Ahmet Helvacioglu, and Shannon Gilmore. (2018). *Hyperprolactinaemia: A Guide for Psychiatrists*. Cambridge: Cambridge University Press.

[Online]   https://cks.nice.org.uk/topics/psychosis-schizophrenia/prescribing-information/monitoring/.

[Online] https://go.drugbank.com/drugs/.

[Online] www.gov.uk/guidance/psychiatric-disorders-assessing-fitness-to-drive.

[Online] www.mind.org.uk/information-support/drugs-and-treatments/antidepressants/side-effects-of-antidepressants/.

[Online] www.nhs.uk/conditions/clinical-trials/.

[Online] www.nhs.uk/conditions/stevens-johnson-syndrome/.

[Online]   www.rcpsych.ac.uk/mental-health/treatments-and-wellbeing/lithium-in-pregnancy-and-breastfeeding.

[Online] www.slam.nhs.uk/media/19073/clozapine.pdf.

[Online] https://slam.nhs.uk/media/18276/lithium.pdf.

[Online]   www.sussexpartnership.nhs.uk/sites/default/files/documents/clozapine_guidance_-_combined_-_dec_15_-_other_medicines_warning_added.pdf.

Peppers, M. (1996). Benzodiazepines for Alcohol Withdrawal in the Elderly and Patients with Liver Disease. *Pharmacotherapy*, 16.

Poels, Eline M. P., Hilmar H. Bijma, Megan Galbally, and Veerle Bergink. (2018). Lithium During Pregnancy and After Delivery: A Review. *International Journal of Bipolar Disorders*, 6 (26).

Sweet, R. A., E. J. Brown, R. G. Heimberg, L. Ciafre, D. M. Scanga, J. R. Cornelius, S. Dube, K. M. Forsyth, and C. S. Holt. (1995). Monoamine oxidase inhibitor dietary restrictions: what are we asking patients to give up? *Journal of Clinical Psychiatry*, 56 (5).

Taylor, P. K. (2015). *The Maudsley Prescribing Guidelines in Psychiatry*. Ney York: Wiley Blackwell.

Yeragani, T. S., Sathyanarayana Rao, and K. Vikram. (2009). Hypertensive Crisis and Cheese. *Indian Journal of Psychiatry*, 51.

Part V

Classification and Assessment

15 Classification

Richard Kerslake

a) Diagnostic Manuals

The main diagnostic manuals:

* International Classification of Diseases (ICD)
* Diagnostic and Statistical Manual of Mental Disorders (DSM)

These manuals are used to *group* psychiatric disorders and *define* them with agreed criteria.

ICD

Managed by the *World Health Organisation*:

* First ICD was published in 1855.
* A categorical system with ten major categories.
* Used for many **general medical** conditions.
* Psychiatric disorders are in *Chapter 5* (of 21 chapters), identified by the code '*F*'.
* Uses an open *alpha-numeric system*, for example, Fxy.zz:

  x = broad category (mood, psychotic, etc.)
  y = specific diagnosis (recurrent depressive disorder)
  zz = additional specifier

* Different versions exist for clinical diagnosis, research, primary care and clinical coding.
* Compared to worldwide diagnostic guidelines, the correlation was good except for diagnosis of personality disorders.
* ICD-10 is the current version in use, with ICD-11 expected after this book has gone to print.

DOI: 10.1201/9781003322573-21

DSM

Produced by the *American Psychiatric Association*:

- Describes *only mental health* disorders.
- *Closed numerical* coding system, for example, xxx.yy.
- One single version exists, which has a *descriptive approach*.
- Does not align with causal theories such as cognitive or genetic models.
- Diagnoses are not hierarchical, accepting comorbidity.
- DSM-V was released in 2013 but is not widely used apart from in the US, where it is referenced for insurance claims.

b) Changes From DSM-IV to DSM-5

Section I describes:

- How chapters are newly organised.
- How the multiaxial system has changed.
- The use of the 'dimensional approach' in Section III.

Section II contains the diagnostic criteria and related reference codes.

The multiaxial system of DSM-IV has been modified, as in Figure 15.1. Clinical syndromes (Axis I), personality disorders (Axis II) and medical conditions

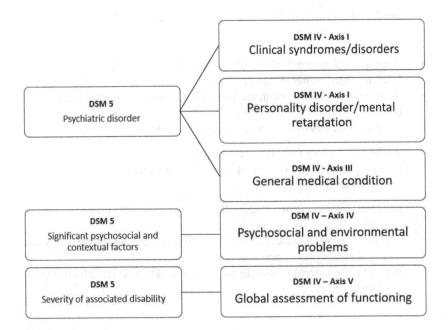

Figure 15.1 Modified DSM axis system

(Axis III) are now classified alongside other under 'psychiatric disorders'. This means that personality disorders are treated with the same significance as other psychiatric disorders.

DSM-5 includes only three axes: psychiatric disorder, significant psychosocial and contextual features and the severity of associated disability.

The classifier 'not otherwise specified (NOS)' has been replaced with 'not elsewhere defined (NED)'.

Schizophrenia subtypes have been removed, as they were considered to be relatively unstable over time.

A new category of autism spectrum disorder has been described, which encompasses what were separately described in DSM-IV as Asperger's syndrome, childhood disintegrative disorder and pervasive developmental disorder.

The term 'mental retardation' has been replaced with 'intellectual disability'.

For the diagnosis of 'depressive disorder', bereavement is no longer an exclusion feature.

Section III outlines the introduction of a 'dimensional approach' to classification which is intended to stimulate further research on the appropriateness on this approach.

c) Approaches to Classification

Classification and diagnosis are not always beneficial to the patient, but there are some definite advantages to this approach:

1. It provides an accepted *standard* for what constitutes a mental health diagnosis.
2. It allows precise *communication* between clinicians about a diagnosis.
3. It helps with the appropriate *prescribing* of medications.
4. It allows *comparable research* between different research teams.
5. It helps research to guide *treatment* on an individual patient. Psychiatry is described as usually *polythetic* in its approach, using a cluster of clinical features rather than a single pathognomonic feature to reach a diagnosis.

The following systems outline the approaches that are possible, sometime incorporating multiple styles, for example, ICD-10 is a categorical and operationalised multi-axial approach.

Categorical Approach

Disorders are clearly separated by definitions, with patients either meeting or not meeting a diagnosis. Diagnoses are therefore easily communicated. This method has *good diagnostic reliability*, as it is easy to understand.

But, this method has *poor validity*. Distinctions between categories may be arbitrary and not always clearly identified in clinical practice. Some patients have features overlapping categories. It is not useful for disorders that are defined as relative to 'normal', such as learning disabilities.

'Multi-axial' systems use separate sets of categories such as chronicity, personality and disability to give an improved clinical representation of the subject.

Dimensional Approach

Aspects of presenting psychopathology are given a score:

- Subject is categorised on varied dimensions.
- More *individualised* interpretation.
- *Better validity.*

This method recognises that diagnostic features can exist to degrees and not as all-or-nothing features. It allows for severity to be better demonstrated. It better accounts for comorbid diagnoses. It has greater power as a research method.

This system is difficult to apply in clinical practice.

Operationalised Approach

Defined clinical criteria are extended to describe *inclusion or exclusion criteria* and features such as duration or relapses.

This takes account *characteristic symptoms*, which are considered relevant but not specific to a diagnosis, for example, low mood, and *discriminating symptoms*, which are more specific, for example, thought insertion.

For example: F31.51 bipolar affective disorder, current episode severe depression with mood incongruent psychotic symptoms.

This system was introduced in DSM-III.

This system can be applied to computerised scoring software.

Hierarchical Approach

If a diagnosis higher up the hierarchical list explains the presentation, then diagnoses further down the list will be refuted. This can *dismiss comorbidity*. Karl Jaspers followed this model with organic disorders at the top of the hierarchy.[1]

ICD-10 has some hierarchy, but the approach is mostly abandoned in the DSM.

A good classification system must demonstrate:

> **Reliability**—measures the degree of agreement on a diagnosis, from two independent assessments, using that system. This can be improved by structured interviews, an index of terminology and an operationalised approach.

Validity—does that system reach the correct diagnosis (usually, compared to a gold standard)?

Face validity—corresponding with current clinical practice.

Predictive validity—corresponding with expected outcomes and treatment response.

Construct validity—corresponding with underlying aetiology and pathophysiology.

Note

1. Stanghellini, G., and T. Fuchs (Eds.). (2013). *One Century of Karl Jaspers' General Psychopathology*. Oxford: Oxford University Press, pp. 185–207.

16 History and Mental State Examination

Richard Kerslake

a) The Psychiatric History

The purpose of the psychiatric history is to:

- Develop a therapeutic alliance—demonstrated to positively affect clinical outcomes at 20 months[1].
- Gather clinical information.
- Formulate and diagnose.
- Agree on a management plan.

The role of empathy in the psychiatric interview cannot be understated. The word is derived from the Greek, translating literally as 'feeling into'. This concept goes beyond sympathy, which is derived from the Greek 'feeling together'. It implies that the clinician has understood the patient's internal world sufficiently that they are able to imagine themselves 'into' the experiences. A history that establishes this depth of understanding will provide an accurate formulation and diagnosis, in which the patient is central.

Techniques to improve the interview:[2]

- Appear relaxed and unhurried.
- Maintain eye contact and minimise note taking.
- Consider factual content as well as verbal/non-verbal indicators of distress.
- Maintain control of the interview for over-talkative patients.

Understanding question styles:

Open questions allow patients to provide a qualitative and expansive answer: *'What can I help you with today?'*

DOI: 10.1201/9781003322573-22

Closed questions can generate specific or factual answers: '*Have you had problems sleeping?*'

Leading questions can guide the patient's answer: '*It sounds as though you've been drinking a lot recently?*'

Compound questions ask multiple about themes in a sentence, which can confuse the patient and clinician: '*Have you been anxious or paranoid recently?*'

Imperative questions will direct a patient on the topic to talk about using a command: '*Tell me more about that incident.*'

Recognised prompts and facilitators include:

Facilitators, which must be genuinely expressed: '*That must have been a very difficult time for you.*'

Reflections, where the observed emotions are named: '*I can see that has made you very worried.*'

Recapitulation can be used to restate the patient's own words as clarification and to summarise.

Active listening using non-verbal gestures can be demonstrated by facial expressions or nodding appropriately.

Pre-verbal communication can express empathy through non-words: '*Uh-huh*' or '*hmmm*'.

Signposting can warn and prepare a patient that '*I need to ask you about some quite sensitive issues now*'.

Sensitive use of **silences** can be useful when a disclosure is anticipated.

Text Box 16.1

Doctor-Patient Styles

Paternalistic/autocratic—the doctor knows best; the doctor decides on treatment; the patient is expected to comply.

Informative—the doctor provides the information, with the patient making the choice alone.

Interpretive—the doctor understands the patient's priorities and supports their participation to reach a shared choice.

Deliberative—the doctor directs the patients to what he sees as their best interest but leaves the decision to the patient.

Text Box 16.2

The Structure of the Psychiatric History

The following is an accepted format for documenting the patient's history.
Name, age, address, who referred, where was patient seen.

Presenting Complaint
Record the patient's own words and/or the words of the referrer.

History of Presenting Complaint
To be presented chronologically where appropriate.

Past Psychiatric History
Diagnoses and treatments.
Admissions including voluntary or under section.
Episodes of harm to self or others—asking about suicide does NOT
increase the risk.

Medication History
Medical and psychiatric, ask about compliance.
Allergies.

Family History
Draw a genogram (Figure 16.1) including parents, siblings and children.
Medical and psychiatric diagnoses should be noted.
Include history of suicide and substance misuse.

Personal History
Pregnancy events and birth events.
Developmental milestones, early life attachments or separations.
Health or emotional events.
Schooling, university and level of attainment.
Occupations and psychosexual history and relationships.

Substance History
Alcohol, recreational and over-the-counter drugs of abuse.

Social History
Accommodation, living circumstances and finances.

Forensic History
Past, present and future plans;
to self, others and property.

Personality Factors
Character, habits and relationship patterns.

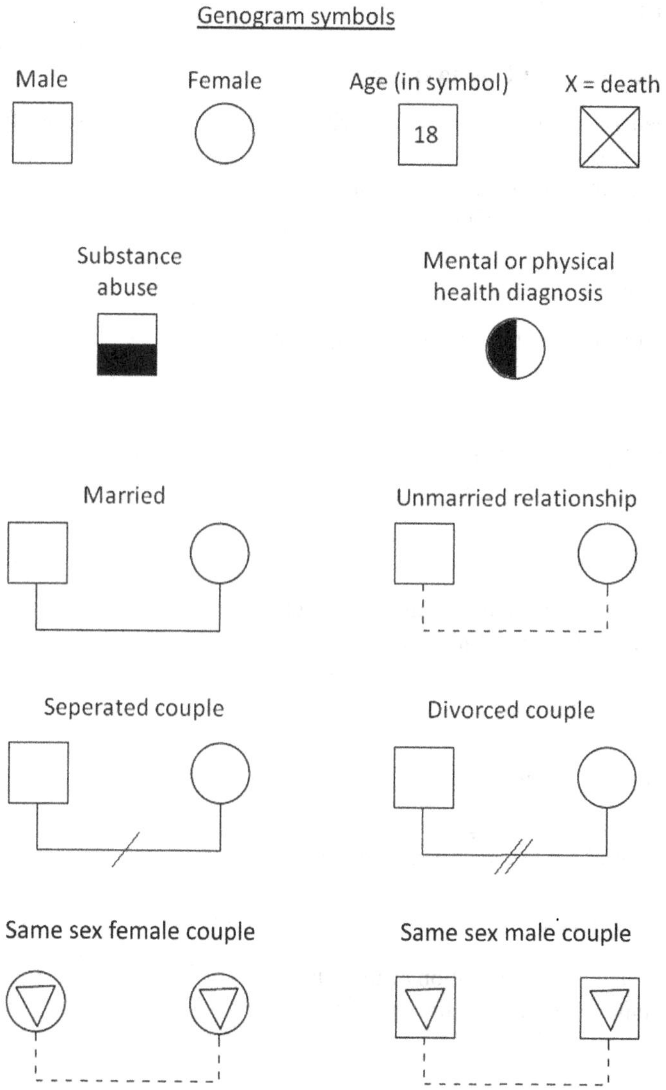

Figure 16.1 Genogram symbols

The **mental state examination** is the psychiatrist's equivalent of a cardio-vascular or respiratory examination. It is an assessment of signs and symptoms (see Chapter 17) *at that specific time.* This can support the presence of a diagnosis or be compared to a past or future examination.

Text Box 16.3

Appearance and Behaviour

General appearance and identifying features, level of self-care, facial expressions
Abnormal movements or posture
Rapport and eye contact

Speech

Rate, volume, tone, prosody and accents

Mood

Subjectively and objectively
Depersonalisation, derealisation

Affect

Consider the quality, range and congruity
Dissociation/incongruity of affect

Suicidal Ideation

Thought Content

Delusion (including the type)
Overvalued ideas, intrusive thoughts

Thought Form

Stream and organisation of thoughts
Comment on formal thought disorder

Perceptions

Auditory, visual, olfactory, gustatory and tactile hallucinations, illusions and distortions

Cognition

Insight

Level of insight, views on diagnosis and treatment

b) Cognitive Function

An in-depth assessment of cognition is most necessary in instances of delirium, dementia and depressive pseudodementia.

The main domains of cognition are covered in the following tests:

The **Mini Mental State Examination**[3] is the most common bedside test of cognition, but it neglects the frontal lobe functions. The follow areas are covered:

Orientation (10 points): Time—name the: year, month, season, date, day
Place—name the: country, county, city/town, building, floor/ward

Registration (3 points) Subject Must Repeat Three Named Items
Attention and Concentration (5 points)
Serial 7s? Spell 'WORLD' backwards or list months in reverse order?
Recall (3 points):
Of three named items.
Language (9 points):
Comprehension, expression and repetition
Further neuropsychological testing for:

Attention—digit span, trail making test
Language—Verbal fluency, Boston naming test
Memory—Weschler memory scale, Ray auditory verbal learning test
Visuospatial skills—Rey-Osterrieth complex figure test
Executive function—Wisconsin card sorting test, Stroop test, Trials B test

The following lobes have established roles in cognitive function:

Frontal lobe (inhibition and abstract concepts):

Abstract Concepts

Proverb interpretation, for example, explain 'every cloud has a silver lining'.
Cognitive estimates, for example, 'how tall is the tallest person'?
Similarities, for example, of a table and a chair; apple and orange?

Response Inhibition

Luria motor test? Go-no go test?

Verbal Fluency

How many animals can be named in 60 seconds?
How many words beginning with F/A/S?

Table 16.1 BMI ranges

<18.5	18.5–24.9	25–29.9	30–39.9	40+
Underweight	Normal range	Overweight	Obese	Morbidly obese

Temporal lobe (largely memory):

Dominant lobe—word recall
Read a sentence? Write a sentence? Recall an address?
Non-dominant—pictorial recall
Recall a drawing?
Bilateral lobes—short-term memory
Recall of address? Recall of named objects?
Bilateral lobes—long-term memory
What school did you go to? What addresses have you lived at?
Semantic memory
Why are the Twin Towers famous? Why was JFK famous?
Working memory
Digit span and reverse digit span test?

Parietal lobe (largely visuospatial):

Dominant lobe—(think *Gerstmann's syndrome*)
Test *calculation, writing, finger recognition* and *L-R orientation*?
Non-dominant lobes—(visuospatial neglect)
Intersecting pentagons, or clock-face drawing?

Bilateral lobes

Recognising object placed in the hand (*asteerognosis*). Recognising
figure drawn in palm (*dysgraphaesthesia*).
BMI = mass (kg)/height^2 (m^2)

BMI ranges are outlined in Table 16.1.

c) The Neurological Examination

The neurological examination and its relevance to psychiatry:
Observe the patient:

Gait

Parkinsonian—festinant shuffling gait with stooped posture and minimal
arm swing.
Cerebellar disease—broad based gait.
Huntington's chorea—'hyperkinetic' gait, jerky, involuntary movements
in all extremities.

Abnormal Movements

Akinesia—absence of control of voluntary muscles.

Bradykinesia—slowness of movement.

Akathisia—subjective feeling of inner restlessness where patient will appear unable to sit still.

Athetosis—continuous stream of slow, flowing writhing movements.

Chorea (basal ganglia disease)—brief, semi-directed, irregular contractions that are not repetitive or rhythmic, but appear to flow from one muscle to the next.

Myoclonus—sudden, involuntary, muscle jerks—not suppressible.

Tic—sudden, repetitive, non-rhythmic, stereotyped movements or vocalisations; are suppressible.

Dystonia—sustained painful muscle contractions—oculogyric (eyes), torticollis (neck).

Tardive dyskinesia—involuntary movements of muscles, often around the face.

Tremor—'pill rolling' in Parkinson's disease, course tremor of lithium toxicity.

Intention tremor—lithium therapy or cerebellar disease.

Hemiballismus—repetitive but varying, *large amplitude* involuntary movements of proximal limbs.

Glasgow Coma scale—orientation, posture or abnormal movements, wasting or fasciculations.

Sit up-squat-stand test—assesses muscle weakness in eating disorders:

1. Patient lies down flat on the floor and sits up without using their hands, if possible; then
2. Patient squats down and rises without using their hands, if possible.

Speech

Dysarthria or dysphasia.

Tone

Cog-wheeling, lead pipe rigidity, spasticity, clonus.

Power and Reflexes

C5–6 = biceps reflex
C7–6 = triceps reflex
C5–6 = supinator
L3–4 = knee
S1–2 = ankle

Babinski sign = up-going plantars in upper motor neuron (UMN) lesions.

Coordination

Finger-nose, dysdiadochokinesia, heel up and down shin.

Sensations

Light touch, pain and temperature, vibration and joint position sense (Figure 16.2).

Cranial Nerves

I = Olfactory—sense of smell.
II = Optic—*AFRO*: visual *A*cuity, *F*ields, pupillary *R*eflexes and *O*ptic disc.

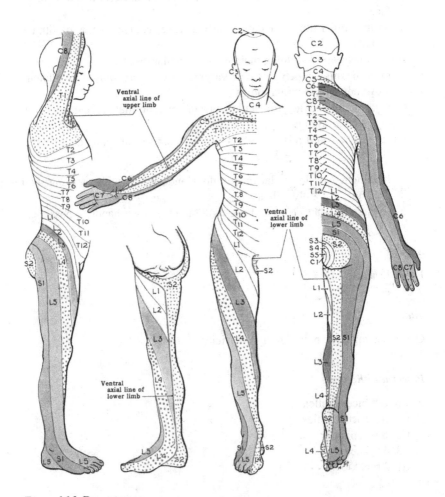

Figure 16.2 Dermatomes

III = Oculomotor, IV = Trochlear, VI = Abducens—eye movements.

V = Trigeminal—sensation of corneal reflex and regions supplied by three divisions; motor function of muscles of mastication.

VII = Facial—sensation of taste over anterior two-thirds of tongue, motor function when baring teeth, raising eyebrows and puffing cheeks.

VIII = Vestibulocochlear—sensation involved in hearing and balance.

IX = Glossopharyngeal and X = Vagus—gag reflex.

XI = Accessory muscle—motor supply to trapezii and sternomastoids.

XII = Hypoglossal—motor supply to tongue muscles.

d) Blood Investigations

Full Blood Count

Chronic alcohol excess—macrocytosis.
Clozapine therapy—agranulocytosis.
Anorexia nervosa—normocytic normochromic anaemia.

Urea + Electrolytes

SSRIs—hyponatraemia.
Bulimia nervosa—hypokalaemia from vomiting.
Anorexia nervosa—hyponatraemia from water loading; hypokalaemia from laxative misuse.

Liver Function Tests

Chronic alcohol use—all parameters raised including gamma glutamyl transferase.
Anorexia nervosa—raised transaminases.

Fasting Glucose or HbA1C

Clozapine or olanzapine—impaired glucose tolerance.

Calcium

Hypercalcaemia—fatigue, depression and confusion. Can be due to lithium and thiazide use.

Glucose

Anorexia—hypoglycaemia.

Endocrine Tests

Depression—exclude hypothyroidism.

Anxiety/mania—exclude hyperthyroidism.
Anorexia nervosa:

- low T3, low/normal T4, normal thyroid stimulating hormone.
- low oestradiol, low luteinising hormone, low follicle stimulating hormone.
- hypercortisolism.
- raised growth hormone.

Prolactin

Antipsychotics—hyperprolactinaemia.

Lipid Profile

Antipsychotics—hypercholesterolaemia.
Anorexia nervosa—hypercholesterolaemia.

Serum Phosphate

Anorexia nervosa and refeeding syndrome—hypophosphatemia.
Bulimia nervosa—hyperphosphataemia.

Lithium Levels

Twelve-hour trough level to check appropriateness of dose.
Random level to check for toxicity.

Arterial Blood Gas

Bulimia nervosa—vomiting leads to metabolic alkalosis; purging leads to metabolic acidosis.

Electrocardiogram (ECG)

Antipsychotics—prolonged Q-T interval.
Cholinesterase inhibitors—arrhythmias.
Anorexia nervosa—arrhythmias, prolonged Q-T interval, non-specific T-wave changes, hypokalaemic changes.

Brain Imaging

First episode psychosis—computed tomography (CT) or magnetic resonance imaging (MRI) brain imaging.

Bone Density Scan

Anorexia nervosa—osteoporosis/osteopenia.

Text Box 16.4

Dementia Screen

Full blood count, urine and electrolytes, liver function tests, ESR/ CRP, glucose, calcium, thyroid function tests, B12 and folate.

Consider chest X-ray and mid-stream urine if delirium is suspected.

Consider cerebrospinal fluid examination if CJD is suspected or the dementia is rapidly progressive.

CT brain—exclude mass lesions, infarction or haemorrhage, normal pressure hydrocephalus.

MRI brain—more sensitive for focal hippocampal atrophy or small vessel disease. Preferred by NICE.

---

e) Specialist Dementia Scans

DaTscan—for Lewy body disease:

Perfusion hexamethylpropyleneamine oxime (HMPAO) single photon emission computed tomography (SPECT) can be used to differentiate frontotemporal dementia from vascular dementia and Alzheimer's disease. Patients with Down syndrome may show similar findings throughout their life, regardless of their dementia status.

Syphilis serology is not routinely requested, instead targeted for at-risk groups.

People with Down syndrome have an increased chance of developing Alzheimer's-type dementia. The following screening tools are more appropriate than the Mini–Mental State Examination (MMSE):

- Dementia Scale for Down Syndrome
- Dementia Questionnaire for Persons with Mental Retardation

f) Delirium

Causes of delirium are outlined in Table 16.2.

Table 16.2 Causes of delirium

Causes of delirium	*Medication causes of delirium*
'I WATCH DEATH'	**'ACUTE CHANGE IN MS'**
*I*nfection	*A*ntibiotics
*W*ithdrawal	*C*ardiac drugs
*A*cute metabolic	*U*rinary incontinence drugs

(Continued)

Table 16.2 (Continued)

Causes of delirium	Medication causes of delirium
Trauma (neck of femur fracture, subdural)	Theophylline
CNS pathology	Ethanol
Hypoxia	Corticosteroids
Deficiencies	H2 blockers
Endocrinopathies	Antiparkinsonian drugs
Acute vascular	Narcotics
Toxins or drugs	Geriatric psychiatric drugs
Heavy metals	ENT (ear, nose and throat) drugs
	Insomnia drugs
	NSAIDs
	Muscle relaxants
	Seizure medicines

g) Eating Disorders

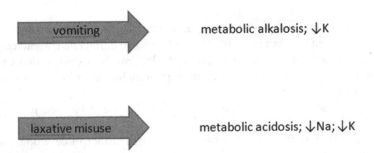

Figure 16.3 Metabolic changes in eating disorders

h) Treatment With Comorbid HIV Infection

Maudsley guidelines for treating psychiatric disorders with comorbid human immunodeficiency virus (HIV)[4]:

Psychosis—atypicals are first line; risperidone is most widely studied.
Delirium—atypicals and low dose short acting benzodiazepines.
Depression—SSRIs, citalopram recommended.
Bipolar—valproate, lamotrigine and gabapentin may be used cautiously; carbamazepine should be avoided.

i) Intelligence Quotient (IQ)

Stanford-Binet Test was the first formalised test with tasks grouped according to *age level*.

Wechsler Adult Intelligence Scale is currently the most widely used IQ test. Uses the *point scale concept* of scoring and *includes a non-verbal* intelligence score.

Raven's Progressive Matrices test *is a non-verbal* test of intelligence measuring 60 items of abstract reasoning.

National Adult Reading Test is used to assess premorbid intelligence in subjects with dementia.

j) Assessment Scales

Self-Rated

Beck Depression Inventory (BDI)—for severity of depression, 21 items, scored 0–3. 14–19 = mild, 20–28 = moderate, 29–63 = severe depression.

Zung Self-Rated Depression Scale (ZSRDS)—for severity of depression, 20 items, score 1–4.

Geriatric Depression Scale (GDS)—screens for depression in elderly, Y/N response to 30 items. 10–19 = mild, 20–30 = severe depression.

Edinburgh Postnatal Depression Scale (EPDS)—*self-report* questionnaire for the last *seven days* scoring *ten items*, scored between *0–3 points*, for females in *primary care* in the post-natal period. It is specific to postnatal depression (PND), ignoring tiredness and irritability, which are not specific indicators of PND. Score: 0–9 = low risk, 10–12 = moderate risk, 13+ = high risk.

Clinician Rated

Montgomery-Asberg Depression Rating Scale (MADRS)—a *ten-item* diagnostic questionnaire designed for the *assessment of treatment effects*.

Young Mania Rating Scale (YMRS)—an *11-item* tool to assess the severity of mania.

Hamilton Depression Rating Scale (HAMD)—a *17- or 21-item multiple choice* questionnaire for rating the *severity* of depression. Items are scored either *3 or 5 points*. Score >24 = severe depression.

Hamilton Anxiety Rating Scale (HAMA)—a *14-item* tool to assess the severity of anxiety.

Yale-Brown Obsessive Compulsive Scale (Y-BOCS)—used to measure the severity of OCD and response to treatment.

Brief Psychotic Rating Scale (BPRS)—assesses *18 or 24 symptom constructs*, over the previous two to three days, that may be reported by the family, scored between *1–7 points*, to *demonstrate change* in overall psychopathology in major disorders, focussing on psychosis. It considers *psychotic* and *affective* symptoms.

Global Assessment of Functioning (GAF)—a single score 0–100 for psychological and social functioning.

Table 16.3 PANSS scale

---

30 items are scored between *1 (absent)* to *7 (extreme)*.

7 'positive' symptoms:	**7 'negative' symptoms:**
Delusions	Blunted affect
Conceptual disorganisation	Emotional withdrawal
Hallucinations	Poor rapport
Hyperactivity	Passive/apathetic social withdrawal
Grandiosity	Abstract thinking difficulties
Suspiciousness/persecutory beliefs	Lacking in spontaneity
Hostility	Stereotyped thinking

16 'general psychopathology' symptoms:

Somatic concerns	Unusual thought content
Anxiety	Disorientation
Guilt feelings	Poor attention
Tensions	Lack of judgement and insight
Mannerisms and posturing	Disturbance of volition
Depression	Poor impulse control
Motor retardation	Preoccupation
Uncooperativeness	Active social avoidance

Clinical Global Impression (CGI)—a measure of illness severity, scored in comparison to other patients with the same diagnosis.

Positive and Negative Symptoms Scale (PANSS)—an observer rated assessment of severity in psychotic illnesses over the last week, as in Table 16.3.

Notes

1. Priebe, S., and T. Gruyters. (1993). The Role of the Helping Alliance in Psychiatric Community Care: A Prospective Study. *Journal of Nervous and Mental Diseases*, 181 (9): 552–557.
2. Goldberg, D. P., J. J. Steele, and C. Smith. (1980). Teaching Psychiatric Interview Techniques to Family Doctors. *Acta Psychiatrica Scandinavica*, 62: 41–47.
3. Folstein, M. F., S. E. Folstein, and P. R. McHugh. (1975). "Mini-mental State". A Practical Method for Grading the Cognitive State of Patients for the Clinician. *Journal of Psychiatric Research*, 12 (3): 189–198.
4. Taylor, D., C. Paton, and S. Kapur. (2009). *The Maudsley Prescribing Guidelines*. London: Informa Healthcare, 10th ed.

17 Psychopathology

Richard Kerslake

Text Box 17.1

Confusion Alert!!

Andrew **Sims** describes form and content as distinct psychopathology.[1] Sims is referring to symptoms form and symptoms content. This is different to thought form and content described in a mental state examination.

Symptoms form—the term used to classify a psychiatric phenomenon. Form is used for diagnostic decisions.

Symptoms content—the subjective colouring of a psychiatric phenomenon.

Content is used for management decisions, for example, a patient describes hearing voices telling them to hang themselves.

The content of the phenomenology is suicidal themes.

The form is auditory hallucinations.

---

a) Thought Disorders

Assessment will consider:

Thought form—are the thoughts being formed appropriately?
Cannot be assessed from behaviour alone; will require the patient to speak.
Insight can be maintained.
The stream and flow of thoughts may also be commented on.
Thought content—what is being thought about?
A subject's behaviour could indicate abnormal thought content.
If delusions are present, insight will not be maintained.

DOI: 10.1201/9781003322573-23

Text Box 17.2

Formal Thought Disorder

Formal Thought Disorder is when thought form is disorganised to a qualifiable degree, for example, loosening of associations, word salad, tangentiality etc.

Formal Thought Disorder implies psychosis.

Formal Thought Disorder can be seen in organic syndromes.

Paralogia = Formal Thought Disorder due to abnormal elements added to normal thought form, for example, tangentiality or flight of ideas.

Alogia = Formal Thought Disorder due to elements lost from normal thought form, for example, thought block or retardation of thoughts.

---

b) Classifying Thought Form

Normal thinking:

Fantasy/dereistic thinking—not goal directed, like daydreaming.

Imaginative thinking—goal directed, imagined abstract concepts, based in possibility.

Rational/conceptual thinking—logical and based in reality.

Disordered thinking:

Normam **Cameron's** characteristics[2]:

Metonymy—imprecise but approximate expressions.

Asyndesis—absence of casual links in speech.

Overinclusion—ideas that are only loosely related are expressed—loss of conceptual boundaries.

Derailment—'entgleisen'—misdirection of the thoughts from their goal—move off track.

Carl **Schneider's** (1930) Five characteristics[3]—SOFDD:

Substitution—of a thought for a less appropriate one.

Omission—a section of thought is missed out from the stream, unnoticed by the subject.

Fusion—direction is lost as thoughts stick together.

Drivelling—meaningful thoughts become deteriorate into muddled senselessness.

Derailment (as explained previously).

Concrete thinking—subject unable to think in the abstract; associated with schizophrenia, fronto-temporal dementia and Asperger's.

Thought block—sudden freeze in the flow of thoughts; associated with psychosis.

Semantic problems that conceptualise thought form:

Clang associations—thoughts are linked through their sounds via punning or rhyming. Usually though first syllables in schizophrenia. Usually through end syllables in mania.

Neologism—made-up words.

Metonyms—word approximations—'walltimer' for 'clock'.

Stock words—using a word or phrases frequently in an idiosyncratic ways where the meaning appears misunderstood.

Paraphasia—non-verbal sounds substitute a words.

Verbal paraphasia—inappropriate words (may be a neologism or metonym) substituted into a sentence.

Literal paraphasia—a phonologically related non-word is substituted into a sentence—meaning will only be understood by the subject.

Text Box 17.3

Mania and Schizophrenia

Mania is associated with:

- Clang associations
- Flight of ideas

Schizophrenia is associated with:

- Derailment
- Loosening of associations
- Poverty of speech

Andreasen, N C (1979)[4]

The following are examples of stream and pace abnormalities that conceptualise thought form.

Flight of ideas implies mania is present:

- Succession of thoughts is rapid.
- Direction and association between each thought is present but hard to follow.
- Clang associations may be noticed.

Retardation of thinking—implies depression—flow of thoughts is noticeably slowed, but remain goal directed. May be accompanied by latency of response and prolonged pauses.

Circumstantiality:

- Slow progress of thoughts, with unnecessary digressions, but will return to the point
- A 'failure of differentiation of the figure ground'.

- Original descriptions associations with temporal lobe (TL) epilepsy.
- Also associated with obsessional personalities.

Tangentiality—subjects thought progression never reaches the point.

Over-inclusive thinking—concepts that are only remotely important are included in the subject's thought process.

Loosening of associations—links between successive thoughts are oblique, without change in the pace that thoughts are expressed.

Perseveration—thought process cannot move beyond the initial concept—associated with clouded consciousness—pathognomonic of organic brain disease—can be demonstrated through repeated motor tasks.

Vorbeireden—'talking past the point'; FTD.

Vorbeigehen—'going past the point'; associated with Ganser syndrome.

Text Box 17.4

Ganser Syndrome

A dissociative syndrome of prisoners providing approximate nonsensical answers to simple questions implying they know the answer is correct. It can be associated with clouding of consciousness with disorientation.

---

c) Explanatory Models

Theory of mind (ToM)—understanding that others have mental processes that may conflict with one's own and will affect interactions. Acute deficiencies of ToM in psychotic episodes may explain FTD.

Dysexecutive deficits may influence FTD—relates to psychosis affecting the frontal lobes and their role in language formation, planning and error monitoring.

Eugen **Bleuler** explained FTD as due to loosening of associations.[5]

Eilhard **Von Domarus** explained FTD as due to loss of deductive reasoning.[6]

Ann **Mortimer** explained FTD as due to impaired semantic memory.[7]

Akataphasia = Emil **Kraepelin's** term for the speech disorders that resulted from FTD.[8]

George **Kelly** measured FTD using 'personal constructs theory'.[9]

Linguistic Studies

Schizophrenic subjects score poorly on word association tests.

Cloze procedure—a speech or text provided with words blanked out. Schizophrenic subjects are less able to predict the missing words.

Reverse Cloze procedure—Schizophrenic subjects are less able to predict the meaning of the whole text.

Type-token ratio—number of different words spoken: total number of words; schizophrenia associated with low type-token ratio, implying poor vocabulary.

Cohesion analysis—schizophrenia associated with using pronouns without prior mention of the subject (less referential ties) and using more connecting words (lexical ties).

d) Classifying Thought Content

Delusions—Frank **Fish** in 1967 provides the conventional descriptions of a false, unshakeable belief that is out of keeping with a subjects social and cultural background.[10]

Kenneth S. **Kendler** (1983) describes dimensions of a delusional experience:[11] conviction, extension (to various spheres of life), disorganisation (level of internal consistency and systematisation), bizarreness (could it be real?), pressure (preoccupations and associated distress), acting on or seeking evidence for. Can be bizarre, very strange and completely implausible; or non-bizarre, a belief that is false but could be possible.

Egosyntonic—in keeping and acceptable with the individual's hopes and goals—the opposite being egodystonic.

Mood congruent—delusions with themes that are consistent with a person's mood states ('the power to make the whole world peaceful in mania', 'the sun will never rise again in depression').

Obsessions—recurrent, intrusive, unwanted and unpleasant thoughts.

Patient can understand obsessions as senseless. Tend to be resisted. Causes distress.

Regarded as one's own thoughts but are considered 'ego-alien' (against their values and desires).

May occur before a compulsive act but not always.

Obsessional slowness can occur as:

- As primary obsessional slowness in severe OCD.
- Secondary to obsessions or depression.
- A compulsion to complete acts 'just right'.

Overvalued ideas—a false belief that preoccupies a person's life but is not held with unshakeable intensity of delusions and often has some reality base.

Associated with paranoid personality disorder, body dysmorphia and anorexia nervosa.

Primary Delusions

Originally conceptualised by Karl **Jaspers**—un-understandable; their cause cannot be reduced to other mental experiences.[12]

Contemporary psychiatry considers primary delusions as arising without identifiable precipitating event[13]:

- Do not carry prognostic significance.
- Tend to be associated with acute stages of psychosis.

Secondary Delusions

Text Box 17.5

Four Types of Primary Delusions

Autochthonous delusions—'out of the blue'; occurring in a sudden moment of delusional knowledge.

Delusional perceptions—a normal perception that is given a delusional meaning (usually self-referential). This is the only first-rank symptom that is a delusion.

Delusional mood—a salient sense that something odd and significant is going on, association with early stages of psychosis.

Is an affective state—would be most correctly described under 'mood' in the mental state examination.

Delusional mood is the only phenomenon that can precede a primary delusion.

Delusional memory—either:

A false memory, often bizarre, is reported as having occurred and being remembered.

Or, a true memory is given a delusional significance.

Secondary delusions arise from abnormal experiences, that is, after an auditory hallucination.

Persecutory delusions—the subject believes they are in imminent danger or harm is intended to them from a specific source. Persecution is recognised as the commonest delusional content.

Morbid jealousy—belief that a partner is being unfaithful. Can be delusional (Othello syndrome) or as an overvalued idea.

Associated with alcoholism.

Has a high potential for violence.

Erotomania—delusion of love. Classical description of De Clérambault's syndrome = female subject believing an older man, usually of higher social standing, is in love with her.

Folie a deux—French for 'madness of two'; shared delusions when the belief is also held by someone close to the subject.

Doppelganger—heautoscopy; seeing oneself at a distance.

Text Box 17.6

Doppelganger[14]

Doppelganger is a cognitive and ideational concept—seeing oneself where nothing is present.
  Different than autoscopy, which is a perceptual phenomenon.
  Different than subjective doubles, where another person is identified as transformed into the subject's self.

Cotard's 'walking corpse' delusions—the subject believes he/she is dead though nihilistic delusions. Associated with severe depression with or without psychotic features and schizophrenia and often more common in the elderly.

Couvade syndrome—conversion symptoms of pregnancy experienced by a husband during a wife's pregnancy. Not held with delusional intensity.

Pseudocyesis—a female subject experiencing symptoms of pregnancy with a negative pregnancy test.

Somatisation—preoccupations with symptoms without a specific diagnosis of concerns.

Hypochondriasis—preoccupations with a serious illness.

Confusingly, there are a group of monosymptomatic hypochondriacal psychoses that do not involve preoccupation with a specific illness:

* Delusions of body odour or halitosis—is by definition a false belief, so there is no identifiable smell.
* Delusion of infestation—Ekbom's syndrome: belief that macroscopic parasites are present on the skin; matchbox sign: patient will bring in a matchbox containing skin scrapings which are supposed to evidence their concerns.
* Delusions of dysmorphia—belief that a part of the body is misshaped or malformed.

Delusion of reference—belief that a coincidence or observed event is of specific personal reference to the self, for example, an advert on a bus.

Ideas of reference—a subjective sense that others are taking specific notice of oneself; associated with paranoid personality disorder.

Thought alienation—a subject's thoughts are experienced as being influenced or controlled by an external agency.

Passivity phenomenon—thought insertion, thought withdrawal and thought broadcasting; part of 'Schneider's First Rank' symptoms.

The predominant underlying feature is disturbance of ego-boundary (where is the edge of the self).

Text Box 17.7

Schneider's First Rank Symptoms

A symptoms cluster—one or more symptoms suggests a diagnosis of schizophrenia, if organic illness is ruled out.

Three Hallucinations

Thought echo—thoughts are heard out loud after they are experienced

Third person auditory hallucination (AH)—talking about the subject

Running commentary on subject's actions

Three Made Phenomena

Made affect—mood/affect controlled by external agency

Made volition—(completed) actions are controlled by external agency

Made impulses—subject's drive or desires are controlled by external agency

Three Thought Phenomena

Thought withdrawal—by external agency

Thought insertion—by external agency

Thought broadcasting/diffusion—thoughts can be known by others as and when they are experienced

Two Isolated Symptoms

Delusional perception

Somatic passivity—body sensations are under control by external agency

This model has provided the basis for the ICD-10 classification of schizophrenia. It is:

NOT a comprehensive list of symptoms of schizophrenia

NOT pathognomonic of schizophrenia, can be seen in other conditions

NOT prognostic

NOT essential for a diagnosis of schizophrenia

Text Box 17.8

Misidentification Syndromes

CaPgRas syndrome—delusional belief that a known **P**erson has been **R**eplaced by an exact double.

Fregoli syndrome—false familiarity of a stranger as a person taking on various disguises. It was named after a French character actor who was good a disguising himself.

Syndrome of subjective doubles—exact double of him/herself exist.

Intermetamorphosis—the subject believes people can fully transform themselves at will into others.

Neuropsychology Theories of Delusions

Attentional bias—paranoia is related to increased recall of and attention to experiences perceived as threatening.

Attributional bias—events which could hypothetically support delusional beliefs are given increasing significance.

Probabilistic reasoning bias—'jumping to conclusions'; in probability experiments, subjects with delusions have been shown to infer false conclusions with more hastily and with less information than controls.

Mentalising bias—subjects with paranoid delusions are more likely to falsely interpret the behaviours and intentions of others—'theory of mind' deficits.

e) Disorders of Speech

Speech may be classified as:

Pressured = rapid, without pauses and 'uninterruptible'
Stilted = overpolite and excessively formal quality
Prosody of speech refers to the patterns of stress and intonation used.
Organic speech disorders

Receptive Dysphasia

Primary sensory dysphasia (Wernicke's)—impaired understanding of spoken word but able to speak fluently.

Pure word deafness—impaired understanding of speech with intact speech, reading and writing. Lesions in dominant temporal lobe.

Table 17.1 Verbigeration

	Speech	Compre-hension	Naming	Repetition	Reading	Writing
Primary sensory dysphasia (Wernicke's)	fluent	absent		absent	absent	absent
Pure word deafness	fluent	absent	intact	absent	intact	intact
Pure word blindness	fluent	intact	intact	intact	absent	intact
Conduction dysphasia	fluent	intact		absent		absent
Nominal dysphasia	fluent	intact	absent	absent		
Primary motor dysphasia (Broca's)	non-fluent			absent		absent
Pure word dumbness	non-fluent	intact		absent	intact	intact

Pure word blindness—impaired reading comprehension with normal speech, writing and understanding of spoken word. Alexia without agraphia.

Conduction dysphasia—repetition of speech and writing is impaired but comprehension alone or expression alone are intact; damage to the arcuate fasciculus (conduction pathway between Wernicke's and Broca's area).

Nominal dysphasia—difficulty in naming with intact ability to describe.

Expressive Dysphasia

Primary motor dysphasia (Broca's)—impaired production of speech and writing with intact comprehension.

Pure word dumbness—difficulty in producing motor speech with intact comprehension and writing. Muscles intact for other purposes.

Pure agraphia—isolated inability to write.

Functional speech disorders

Stuttering and stammering

Mutism—akinetic/elective/selective

Vorbeireden

Neologisms

Logoclonia—senseless repetition of syllables

Echolalia—senseless repetition of words or phrases; associated with dementia and mental retardation

Verbigeration—stereotypes and meaningless repetition of words or syllables, as outlined in Table 17.1.

f) Disorders of Memory

Can be classified into:

* Sensory memory—automatic but dissipates within seconds; information received by the five senses is rapidly graded as useful or not.

Iconic = visual; echoic = auditory; haptic = touch.
   If deemed relevant, the information is stored in:

* Short-term (working) memory—lasts seconds to minutes. Used to address task at hand. Sensitive to brain disorders for example, Alzheimer's disease.
* Long-term memory—encoded through rehearsal. Believed to have unlimited an unlimited storage capacity. 'Resilient to attack', allowing for recall of events from the past.

The sieve model shows each stage of memory (Figure 17.1):

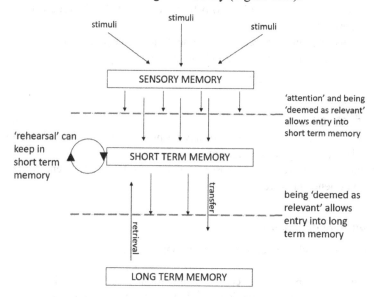

Figure 17.1 Sieve model of memory

Memory can be classified into (Figure 17.2):

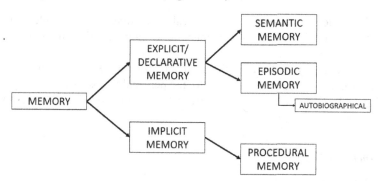

Figure 17.2 Memory classification

- Explicit/declarative memory—requires conscious storage and retrieval.
- Semantic memory—abstract knowledge, facts that are independent of context—dates of World War I.
- Episodic—recalling specific events, context specific.
- Autobiographical—recall of events experienced in the past.
- Flashbulb memories—a unique episodic memory with a strong emotional significance attached.

Implicit Memory

No conscious recall is required. Mostly used in motor tasks requiring procedural memory.

Demonstrated when repeating a task leads to better performance.

Associated with cerebellum and basal ganglia.

Amnesia—loss of memory.

Recognition:

Déjà vu—'already seen'—sense of having previously experienced and event which is happening for the first time.

Jamais vu—'never seen'—absence of familiarity for an event which has been experienced before.

Falsification of Memory

- Confabulation—occurring in clear consciousness.

'Filling in the gaps' without conscious intention to deceive. Subject is usually unaware that the information is false, despite incontrovertible evidence.

Association with organic cause, classically described in Korsakoff's amnesia.

Association with lethologica—inability to recall names or proper nouns.

- Pseudologia fantastica—'pathological' lying, fluent and plausible, usually with a grandiose flavour. Confabulation without organic pathology.[15]

'Falsification entirely disproportionate to any discernible end in view[16]'.

Association with dissocial and histrionic personality disorders.

When faced with contrary incontrovertible evidence, subjects will often admit to lying.

Dissociative Fugue

- Wandering episode.
- Narrowing of consciousness.

- Retrospective amnesia for the episode.
- Subjects report loss of identity during the episode.

Pseudodementia

- Depression preceding cognitive deficits.
- Onset of cognitive deficits is usually clearly identifiable.
- Diurnal variation (early morning worsening) of cognition may be noted.
- Answers are often 'I don't know' rather than the minimising of ignorance seen in true dementias.

The Clifton Assessment Procedure for the Elderly (CAPE) is a hospital and community tool used to assess quality of life, cognitive and physical deficits

g) Disorders of Mood and Affect

Mood is the subjective experience of a pervasive and sustained emotional state.

Fish (2007) emphasises that an assessment of mood should identify intensity, duration, fluctuations and the patient's own descriptive words (See endnote 10).

Affect is the patient's observed emotional responses at that time. Descriptions should include the quality and the range.

Affective qualities:

Flat—(almost) absence of emotional expression.

Blunted—markedly reduced intensity in emotional expression, but not absent.

Restricted/constricted—narrower range of emotional expression than would be expected.

Labile—brief, excessive fluctuations in emotional expression.

Mixed state—features of depression and mania concurrently.

Kraepelin's description of various mixed states is described in Table 17.2. These are simplified to:

Dysphoric mania—full mania with some depressive symptoms.

Depressive mixed states—full depression with some manic symptoms.

Also recognised is agitated depression—full depression with psychomotor agitation.

Anhedonia—inability to derive pleasure from meaningful activities that are usually perceived as pleasant.

- Physical, for example, eating, physical touch.

Table 17.2 Kraepelin mixed states[17]

	Mood	*Will (volition)*	*Thought process*
Manic stupor	elevated	decreased	decreased
Depressive mania	depressed	increased	Increased
Excited depression	depressed	decreased	increased
Depression with flight of ideas	depressed	increased	decreased
Mania with poverty of thought	elevated	increased	decreased
Inhibited mania	elevated	decreased	increased

• Associated with negative symptoms of schizophrenia.
• Social, for example, interpersonal experiences and conversations.
• Associated with depression.

Alexithymia—subject has an absence of vocabulary for emotions—unable to describe their mood. The classical description identifies accompanying features:

• Diminution of fantasy.
• Reduced symbolic thinking.
• Literal thinking focussed on detail.
• Recognition of one's own feelings is difficult.
• Differentiating body sensations and emotional states is difficult.
• A sense of a 'robot-like' existence.

Associations are recognised with somatoform 'mind-body' disorders and depression.

Depersonalisation—subject feels as if they are unreal, no-longer like a person; the 'as if' quality is important, as this is not a delusion.

• An unpleasant and subjective experience.
• Insight is preserved.
• Usually for a discrete time period (minutes to hours).
• Association with depression most commonly; also includes anxiety, temporal lobe epilepsy and dissociative states.
• Can be experienced as pleasant in recreational substance use, fatigue and meditation.

Derealisation—when the 'as if not real' sensation is applied to subject's environment. Often happens with depersonalisation.

Desomatisation—depersonalisation isolated to a body part.

Deaffectualisation—inability to feel any emotions—an extreme form of anhedonia, beyond loss of pleasure.

Possession states—dissociative 'trance' experience where subject experiences loss of control over their actions and loss of awareness and personal identity. Culturally acceptable in some countries, often with religious associations.

Lycanthropy—possession state where subject experiences being transformed into an animal, usually a wolf.

'Near death experiences'—encompasses autoscopy, out of body and transcendental experiences. Feeling of 'impending ego dissolution' associated with LSD use.

h) Disorders of Perception

Illusions = the altered perceptions of a stimulus.

Complete illusion—missing information is filled in to make sense of a stimulus; tends to occur when not focussing attention.

Affect illusion—the stimulus is affected by mood state, for example, seeing shapes when walking alone in the dark.

Pareidolic illusions—an unrelated stimulus becomes organised into a familiar image, for example, seeing clouds that look like animals; tend to occur with focussed attention.

Synaesthesia—experiencing a sensation from stimulation of an alternative sensory modality, for example, experiencing colour as a smell.

Dysmegalopsia—difficulty identifying the size of objects, for example, micropsia or macropsia.

Hallucinations—a perception where there is no stimulus.

First person auditory—hearing own words aloud 'gedanelautwerden' or 'echo de la pensée'.

Second person auditory—voice is addressing the subject directly.

Third person auditory—voice(s) talking about the subject.

Extracampine—heard from beyond a distance that is physically possible.

Visual—often represent organic pathology, for example, delirium, temporal lobe epilepsy.

Lilliputian—images of small people are seen, for example, Lewy-body dementia.

Gustatory—hallucinations of taste.

Olfactory—hallucinations of smell.

Tactile— 'haptic' hallucinations of touch.

Kinaesthetic—sense of limbs or muscles being moved or manipulated.

Functional—at the same time as a real stimulus in the same modality, for example, hearing angels singing whilst the shower is running.

Reflex—occur following a stimulus in another modality.

Hypnopompic—upon waking.

HypnaGogic—upon Going to sleep.

Text Box 17.9

Catatonia

A state of apparent unresponsiveness to external stimuli in a subject who appears to be alert.

Not to be confused with cataplexy—sudden loss of muscle tone, usually in response to a sudden emotional stimulus such as laughing or a fright.

Not to be confused with catalepsy, described later, which is a feature of catatonia.

The Bush-Francis Catatonia Rating Scale provides some descriptions of associated features.

Posturing/catalepsy—spontaneous maintenance of posture, including mundane, for example, sitting or standing for long periods without reacting.

Echopraxia—mimicking of examiner's movements.

Stereotypy—repetitive non-goal directed motor activity, for example, finger-play, repeatedly touching, patting or rubbing self; abnormality not inherent in act but in frequency.

Mannerisms—odd, purposeful movements (hopping or walking tiptoe, saluting passers-by or exaggerated caricatures of mundane movements); abnormality inherent in act itself.

Rigidity—maintenance of a rigid posture despite efforts to be moved, excluded if cog-wheeling or tremor present.

Negativism—apparent motiveless resistance to instructions or attempts to move/examine patients. Contrary behaviour; does exact opposite of instructions.

Waxy flexibility—during reposturing of patient, patient offers initial resistance before allowing himself to be repositioned, similar to that of bending a candle.

Automatic obedience—exaggerated cooperation with examiner's request or spontaneous continuation of movement requested.

Mitgehen—'anglepoise lamp' arm raising in response to light pressure of finger despite instructions to the contrary.

Gegenhalten—resistance to movement which is proportional to strength of the stimulus; appears automatic rather than wilful.

Ambitendency—patient appears 'motorically stuck' in indecisive hesitant movement.

Stupor—extreme hypoactive, immobile, minimally responsive to stimuli.

Notes

1. Oyebode, F. (2008). *Sims' Symptoms in the Mind: An Introduction to Descriptive Psychopathology*. 4th ed. Philadelphia, PA: Saunders Elsevier.
2. Cameron, N. (1944). Experimental Analysis of Schizophrenic Thinking. In J. S. Kasanin (Ed.), *Language and Thought in Schizophrenia*. New York, NY: The Norton Library.
3. Schneider, C. (1930). *Die Psychologie der Schizophrenen*. Leipzig: Georg Thieme.
4. Andreasen, N. C. (1979). Thought, Language, and Communication Disorders: I. Clinical Assessment, Definition of Terms, and Evaluation of Their Reliability. *Archives of General Psychiatry*, 36 (12): 1315–1321.
5. Peralta, V. and M. J. Cuesta. (2011). Eugen Bleuler and the Schizophrenias: 100 years After. *Schizophrenia Bulletin*, 37 (6): 1118–1120.
6. Williams, E. B. (1964). Deductive Reasoning in Schizophrenia. *The Journal of Abnormal and Social Psychology*, 69 (1): 47.
7. McKay A. P., P. J. McKenna, P. Bentham, A. M. Mortimer, A. Holbery, and J. R. Hodges. (1996). Semantic Memory is Impaired in Schizophrenia. *Biological Psychiatry*, 39: 929–937.
8. Jerónimo, J., T. Queirós, E. Cheniaux, and D. Telles-Correia. (2018). Formal Thought Disorders–Historical Roots. *Frontiers in Psychiatry*, 9: 572.
9. Kelly, G. A. (1970). A Brief Introduction to Personal Construct Theory. *Perspectives in Personal Construct Theory*, 1: 29.
10. Casey, P., and B. Kelly. (2019). *Fish's Clinical Psychopathology: Signs and Symptoms in Psychiatry*. Cambridge: Cambridge University Press.
11. Kendler, K. S. (1983). Overview: A Current Perspective on Twin Studies of Schizophrenia. *American Journal of Psychiatry*, 140 (11): 1413–1425.
12. Walker, C. (1991). Delusion: What did Jaspers Really Say? *The British Journal of Psychiatry*, 159 (S14): 94–103.
13. Sadock, B. J., and V. A. Sadock. (2008). *Kaplan & Sadock's Concise Textbook of Clinical Psychiatry*. Philadelphia: Lippincott Williams & Wilkins.
14. Damas Mora, J. M. R., F. A. Jenner, and S. E. Eacott. (1980). On Heautoscopy or the Phenomenon of the Double: Case Presentation and Review of the Literature. *British Journal of Medical Psychology*, 53 (1): 75–83.
15. Healy, W., and M. T. Healy. (1915). *Pathological Lying, Accusation, and Swindling: A Study in Forensic Psychology* (No. 1). Little, Brown and Co.
16. Griffith, Ezra E. H., Madelon Baranoski, and Charles C. Dike. (1 September 2005). Pathological Lying Revisited. *Journal of the American Academy of Psychiatry and the Law*, 33 (3): 342–349.
17. Maina, G., N. Bertetto, F. Domene Boccolini, G. Di Salvo, G. Rosso, and F. Bogetto. (2013). The concept of mixed state in bipolar disorder: From Kraepelin to DSM-5. *Journal of Psychopathology*. 19: 287–295.

18 Diagnosis and ICD-10 Classification Codes

Richard Kerslake

a) ICD-10 vs. DSM-IV

ICD-10 has:
A single axial version of psychiatric diagnoses in Chapter V.
A multi-axial version divided into:

Axis 1—the mental disorder (including personality disorder and mental handicap)
Axis 2—the degree of disability
Axis 3—current psychosocial problems

DSM-IV uses five axes:

Axis I—clinical disorders
Axis II—personality disorders/mental retardation
Axis III—general medical conditions
Axis IV—psychosocial and environmental problems
Axis V—global assessment of functioning

For a diagnosis of schizophrenia, ICD-10 requires a one-month duration of symptoms. DSM-IV requires six months' duration.

DSM no longer uses the tradition's psychoses-neuroses differentiation, whereas ICD-10 maintains F40 neurotic disorders.

ICD-10 classification codes and diagnoses are presented in the following sections

b) F00—F09 Organic, Including Symptomatic, Mental Disorders

Dementia is defined as presenting evidence of:

1. Decline in memory—usually learning of new verbal and non-verbal information—mild, moderate and severe.

DOI: 10.1201/9781003322573-24

2. Decline in other cognitive abilities, for example, judgement and planning—mild, moderate severe, in clear consciousness—no delirium, declining emotional control or social behaviour for at least six months.

F00 Dementia in Alzheimer's Disease

Criteria for dementia is met without evidence for a central (e.g., vascular disease or Parkinson's disease) or systemic cause (e.g., hypothyroidism) being identified.

N.B., the ICD-10 diagnosis does not require evidence of excessive neurofibrillary tangles and neuritic plaques, but these are considered as confirmatory if found post-mortem.

Five A's are supportive to the diagnosis:

Amnesia, **A**phasia, **A**gnosia, **A**praxia, **A**ssociated (behavioural changes, delusions and hallucinations).

Alzheimer's disease is characterised as having a gradual onset in later life and shows progressive deterioration.

Single-photon emission computerised tomography (SPECT) imaging demonstrates temporal and parietal hypoperfusion in subjects with Alzheimer's disease.

Text Box 18.1

Risk Factors for Alzheimer's Disease

Age	Family history
Head trauma	Hypertension
Heart Disease	Diabetes
CVA	Hypercholesterolaemia
Females	Low educational achievement

F01 Vascular Dementia

Criteria for dementia is met when:

Deficits in higher cortical functions are not equal, for example, poor memory with mild decline in reasoning, etc.

Evidence of focal brain damage demonstrated by neurological examination.

Significant cerebrovascular disease identified by history, examination or tests.

Recognised subtypes = multi-infract, subcortical and mixed.

Vascular dementia is characterised as sudden onset, usually after a cerebral event and having a stepwise progression.

F02 Dementia in Other Diseases Classified Elsewhere

Dementia in Pick's disease (fronto-temporal dementia):

Slow and steady deterioration with frontal lobe involvement identified by two or more of emotional blunting, coarsening of social behaviour, disinhibition or aphasia.

Focal atrophy with knife-blade appearance on brain imaging.

Lewy body dementia is characterised as presenting with fluctuations in cognitive impairment, hallucinations, sensitivity to neuroleptic with rigidity/stiffness and falls.

Dementia in Parkinson's disease if Parkinsonian symptoms have been present for 12 months before the onset of dementia.	vs.	Dementia with Lewy bodies if motor and cognitive symptoms develop within 12 months of each other.

Cortical vs. Subcortical Dementia

A comparison of clinical presentations; this has contested validity.

Cortical Dementia—Grey Matter

Impaired language, memory, executive and visuospatial functions.

Alzheimer's, fronto-temporal dementia, Creutzfeldt-Jakob disease.

Subcortical Dementia—White Matter

Features: personality changes, mood disturbances and movement disorders.

Conditions: Dementias of Parkinson's, Huntington's, Binswanger's and Wilson's diseases, AIDS and progressive supranuclear palsy.

Text Box 18.2

Wilson's Disease 'Hepatolenticular Degeneration'

Failure to excrete copper leads to:

—deposits in brain, liver and Kayser-Fleischer rings in the iris
—degeneration of the lenticular nucleus
—dystonia, tremor or rigidity; behavioural changes; dementia

This condition displays autosomal recessive inheritance through the ATP7B gene, leading to low serum ceruloplasmin and total serum copper.

Coded in ICD-10 under 'diseases of the nervous system G00-G99':

G10 Huntington's Disease (Figure 18.1)

- Autosomal dominant inheritance—CAG repeats.
- Progressive chorea and dementia in the fourth/fifth decade of life and psychiatric manifestations.

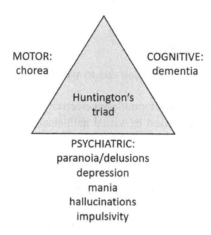

Figure 18.1 Huntington's triad

- Juvenile variant usually involves ++CAG repeats; presentation may include seizures, ataxia, dementia and chorea.

G23.1 Progressive Supranuclear Palsy

A neurodegenerative disorder, presents with balance loss/falls, ophthalmoplegia and memory impairment.
    Similar features to Parkinson's disease, but no tremor.

F05 Delirium, Not Induced by Alcohol and Other Psychoactive Substances

Clouding of consciousness

    AND **D**isturbed cognitions (impaired recall OR disorientation)
    AND **D**isturbed in psychomotor activity
    AND **D**isturbed sleep-wake cycle
    AND **E**vidence of organic pathology is responsible for C+D+D+D
    AND **F**luctuating symptoms with rapid onset

c) F10—F19 Mental and Behavioural Disorders Due to Psychoactive Substance Use

F10—Alcohol

Intoxication: disinhibition, euphoria, skin flushing, slurred speech, ataxia, impaired decision-making ability, nausea and vomiting.
    Withdrawal (*can be fatal*): Anxiety and psychomotor agitation, tremor, nausea and vomiting, seizures, autonomic instability, delirium tremens.

Text Box 18.3

Delirium Tremens (DTs)

(DTs) = rapid onset of confusion due to withdrawal of chronic alcohol consumption.

Global confusion with autonomic hyperactivity (tachycardia and fever).

Historically characterised by visual hallucinations of pink elephants (Figure 18.2).

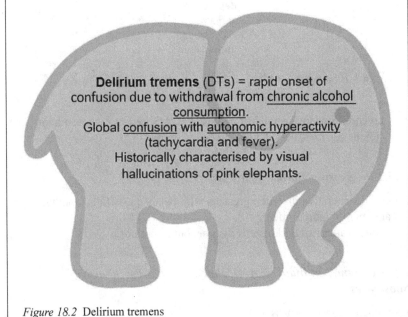

Delirium tremens (DTs) = rapid onset of confusion due to withdrawal from chronic alcohol consumption.
Global confusion with autonomic hyperactivity (tachycardia and fever).
Historically characterised by visual hallucinations of pink elephants.

Figure 18.2 Delirium tremens

F11—Opioids

Intoxication: pupillary constriction, euphoria, drowsiness, constipation, vomiting, respiratory depression.

Withdrawal: *is not fatal.*

Early—muscle pains, sweating, yawning, gastrointestinal (GI) discomfort, runny nose; late—pupillary dilation, vomiting, piloerecetion, diarrhoea.

F12—Cannabinoids

Intoxication: euphoria, intensified sensory experience, conjunctival redness, anxiety, paranoia.

Withdrawal: irritability, reduced appetite, insomnia.

F14—Cocaine

Intoxication: euphoria, agitation, insomnia, pupillary dilation, psychosis, tachycardia, hypertension.

Withdrawal: agitation, dysphoria, depressed mood, fatigue, vivid dreams, hypersomnia.

It is also useful to know the effects of:

MDMA (Ecstasy)

Intoxication: euphoria, enhanced sociability, thermodysregulation and sweating, jaw clenching.

Withdrawal: depression, depersonalisations, derealisation.

Hallucinogens

Intoxication: perceptual distortions, euphoria and dysphoria, tachycardia, sweating.

Withdrawal: no withdrawal syndrome recognised.

Ketamine

Intoxications: euphoria, dissociation, ataxia, perceptual distortions, reduced conscious level.

Withdrawal: no withdrawal syndrome recognised.

The clinical conditions associated with substance use are defined as:

Acute Intoxication

A transient condition.

* Disturbances in level of consciousness, cognition, perception, affect or behaviour.
* Usually related to dose levels.

Harmful Use

Causing 'actual' damage to physical (hepatitis from intravenous drug use) or mental (depression from alcohol) health; should not be diagnosed if dependence syndrome, a psychotic disorder or another specific form of substance related disorder is present.

Dependence Syndrome

A cluster of physiological, behavioural and cognitive phenomena; characteristic feature is when desire to take the substance is strong and sometimes overpowering.

ADDICcT

Activities and alternative interests are neglected:

Dependence physical effect of 'tolerance'—increased doses are required to achieve the effects.

Dependence physical effect of 'withdrawal'—when substance use has ceased or been reduced.

Intrapersonal consequences from persisting with substance use despite harmful physical and mental health consequences.

Compulsion to take the substance.

Controlling difficulties with the onset and offset of substance-taking.

Time consuming or 'narrowing of the repertoire' describing a tendency to drink alcoholic drinks in the daily patterns regardless of social constraints that determine appropriate drinking behaviour.

Withdrawal State

Withdrawal state is a cluster of symptoms due to withdrawing a substance after repeated and prolonged use; onset and course is time-limited; may be complicated by convulsions.

N.B., withdrawal symptoms can be induced by conditioned/learned stimuli in the absence of immediately preceding substance use.

Urine drug screening, and the length of time that substances can be detected, is outlined in Table 18.1.

Table 18.1 Detection periods in urine drug screening[1]

These are approximations and vary between individuals, dosage and length of action.	
Alcohol	7–12 hours
LSD	1 day
Cocaine	6–8 hours
Cocaine metabolites	2–4 days
Amphetamines/MDMA	48 hours
Cannabis (single use)	3 days
Codeine	48 hours
Heroin/morphine	36–72 hours
Methadone	3 days
Cannabis (single use)	3 days
Lorazepam (intermediate acting)	5 days
Phencyclidine (PCP)	8 days
Diazepam (long acting)	10 days
Cannabis (heavy use)	10–30 days

Kaplin & Sadock—concise textbook of psychiatry[2]

d) F20—F29 Schizophrenia, Schizotypal and Delusional Disorder

F20 Schizophrenia

A single core symptom, or at least two secondary symptoms, present for greater than one month:
Core symptoms
Thought withdrawal, insertion, broadcasting or echo.
Hallucinations of voices giving running commentary or discussing the person or originating from a body part.
Delusions of control, influence, passivity or delusional perception.
Secondary symptoms
Thought form has breaks or interpolations—incoherence or irrelevant speech.
Hallucinations in any sensory modality, that are persistent and accompanied by fleeting delusions.
Catatonic features.
Negative symptoms.

Subtypes of Schizophrenia

F20.0 Paranoid Schizophrenia

- Delusions (not necessarily persecutory) and hallucinations (usually auditory) are the prominent features.
- Thought disorder and negative symptoms are less prominent.
- This is the most common subtype.

Hebephrenic Schizophrenia

- Symptoms should be observed for three months.
- Prominent symptoms are thought disorder with loosening of associations and disorganised behaviour characterised by inappropriate and fatuous giggling and odd mannerisms.
- Onset in adolescents with a progressive course leading to rapid development of negative symptoms, social incapacitation and poor self-care.
- Recovery from the first episode is considered rare.
- DSM-IV recognises this subtype as disorganised schizophrenia.

Simple Schizophrenia

- Symptoms should be present for at least 12 months.
- Prominence of negative symptoms—socially withdrawn, poor planning and initiation and limited emotional reactivity.

- Delusions and hallucinations are not prominent, often absent.
- The course is often early onset in teenage years, with a progressive decline, leading to marked social drift. The prognosis is poor.

Schizophrenia subtypes compared between ICD and DSM

ICD-10 schizophrenia subtypes	DSM schizophrenia subtypes
F20.0 Paranoid schizophrenia F20.1 Disorganized schizophrenia F20.2 Catatonic schizophrenia F20.3 Undifferentiated schizophrenia F20.4 Post-schizophrenic depression F20.5 Residual schizophrenia F20.6 Simple schizophrenia F20.8 Other schizophrenia F20.9 Schizophrenia, unspecified	DSM-V no longer defines subtypes of schizophrenia due to their 'limited diagnostic stability, low reliability, poor validity, and little clinical utility'.[3] DSM-IV defines paranoid, disorganised, catatonic, undifferentiated and residual subtypes.

F22 Persistent Delusional Disorder

Symptoms lasting longer than three months:

Delusions make up (almost) the entirety of the psychopathology.
Delusions must be personal, beyond subcultural.
Depression may be present, provided it doesn't exclude the experience of delusions.
Exclusion—no organic brain disease, infrequent hallucinations, no first rank symptoms of schizophrenia.

F23 Acute and Transient Psychotic Disorder

Acute onset—lasting between two weeks and one month:
An acute stressor must be identified.

F23.0 Acute polymorphic psychotic disorder without symptoms of schizophrenia—acute onset, less than two weeks, where hallucination or delusion are markedly variable, changing type and intensity from day to day
F23.1 Acute polymorphic psychotic disorder with symptoms of schizophrenia
F23.2 Acute schizophrenia-like psychotic disorder
F25 Schizoaffective disorder—symptoms of schizophrenia and affective disorder are present simultaneously. Symptoms of schizophrenia and affective disorder are not experienced as separate episodes.

What Is Schizophrenia?

Schizophrenia is a psychotic disorder characterised by a collection of positive symptoms (delusions, hallucinations and thought disorder), negative symptoms (7 As) and behaviour deterioration with social sequelae (Figure 18.3).

It occurs in clear consciousness.

Onset is usually in adolescents, and if untreated, schizophrenia is a progressive disorder deteriorating in a linear or stepwise fashion.

The seven As of negative symptoms of schizophrenia: Alogia, Avolition, Apathy, Affective flattening, Anhedonia, Asociality and Attentional impairment.

Difficulties in defining schizophrenia occur on the individual level when clinicians try to agree on what is not schizophrenia. This has led to a breadth of literature on the subject.

Eugen **Bleuler**[5] first described schizophrenia in 1911.

Primary symptoms we described as manifestations of the organic process of the disease: ambivalence, autism, disturbance of affect and loosening of associations.

Secondary symptoms were described as manifestations of the psychic process: delusions, hallucinations, mannerisms and catatonia.

High levels of 'expressed emotions' (EE) in families are associated with increased relapse rates of schizophrenia.[6]

Features of high EE measured by the Camberwell Family Interview (see endnote 4):

* Hostility—negative attitude directed at the patient.
* Emotional over-involvement—over-protectiveness/self-sacrifice, excessive use of praise or blame by a family member towards the patient.

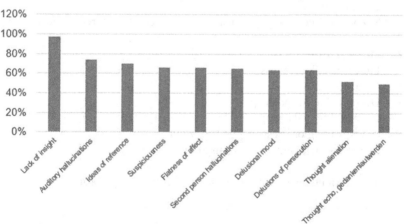

Figure 18.3 Most common symptoms of schizophrenia[4]

- Critical attitudes—combinations of hostile and emotional over-involvement.

e) F30—F39 Mood (Affective) Disorders

F30 Manic Episode

Must be a single episode with no previous affective episodes.

Symptoms for seven days, fewer if requiring hospitalisation. Distinctly abnormal level of elevated mood or irritability.

AND interference in personal functioning in daily living of at least three areas (or four if the mood is irritable):

- Physical restlessness
- Pressured speech
- Flight of ideas
- Loss of normal social inhibitions
- Decreased need for sleep
- Grandiosity
- Distractibility
- Reckless or foolhardy spending, enterprises or other behaviour
- Marked sexual indiscretions

AND not attributable to substance use or other more appropriate diagnosis.

F30.0 Hypomania

Symptoms for four days leading to interference, but not complete disruption, with work:

Elevated or irritable mood

AND notable increase in physical or mental activity in three or more areas:

- Physical restlessness
- Increased talkativeness
- Distractibility
- Decreased need for sleep
- Increased sexual energy
- Overspending or irresponsible behaviour
- Increased sociability or over-familiarity

AND not attributable to substance use or other more appropriate diagnosis.

DSM-V states hypomania occurs without interfering with occupational or social functioning.

F30.1 Mania, without psychotic features
F30.2 Mania, with psychotic features:
Criteria for mania is met
AND delusions or hallucinations are present

F31 Bipolar Affective Disorder

A disorder of two or more authenticated affective episodes, either hypomanic/manic and/or severe depressive episode. Has a tendency for remission and recurrence.

DSM-V subtypes:

Type I—one or more authenticated manic episodes; depression is common but *not necessary* for the diagnosis.
Type 2—one or more hypomanic episodes; a major depressive episode *is necessary* for the diagnosis.

Cyclothymia—hypomanic episodes with depression that doesn't reach criteria for a major depressive episode.

Text Box 18.4

Rapid cycling Bipolar Affective Disorder

Rapid cycling: ♀ > ♂
Defined as four or more affective episodes per year.
Prevalence of 10–20% of bipolar diagnoses.
Tends to develop later in the course of bipolar.
Associated with earlier age of diagnosis.
Increase risk of suicide (inconsistent finding).
More treatment resistant.
Associated with:
Medical factors—thyroid dysfunction, subarachnoid haemorrhage, strokes, multiple sclerosis, propranolol, antidepressants, levodopa, cyproheptadine.
Significant life events.
Alcohol.

F32 Depressive Episode

Core features: depressed mood, loss of interest and enjoyment and reduced energy or increased fatigability.

Other features can be divided into:

Biological
Reduced concentration and attention
Disturbed sleep, for example, early morning wakening

Diminished appetite
Decreased libido
Psychological
Reduced self-esteem and self-confidence
Ideas of guilt and unworthiness
Bleak and pessimistic views of the future
Thoughts of self-harm or suicide

Features should be present for the majority of the time for a minimum of two weeks.

F32.0 Mild Depressive Episode

At least two core features and two other features will be present, with difficulty in continuing social or work functioning, but not ceased completely.

F32.1 Moderate Depressive Episode

Two or three core features and at least three other features will be present, often to a more marked degree, with considerable difficulty in continuing with social, work or domestic activities.

F32.2 Severe depressive episode without psychotic symptoms—all three core features and at least four other features will be present with severe intensity, with considerable distress or agitation, unless retardation is a feature and unable to continue with social, work or domestic activities.

F32.3 Severe depressive episode with psychotic symptoms—as for F32.2 but for F32.3, accompanied by delusions, hallucinations or depressive stupor. Delusions are usually mood-congruent: related to sin, poverty or imminent disasters.

F33 Recurrent Depressive Disorder

Repeated episodes of depression as specified in depressive episode, without any episodes of that fulfil the criteria of mania.

F34.0 Cyclothymia

Persistent instability of mood, involving numerous periods of mild depression and mild elation, not fulfilling the criteria for manic episode or depressive episode.

F34.1 Dysthymia

A chronic depression of mood which does not currently fulfil the criteria for recurrent depressive disorder.

George **Brown** and Tirril **Harris'** 1978 aetiological study of depression identified four 'vulnerability factors' in women:[7]

- With three or more children at home.
- Lacking intimacy with their partner.
- Lacking employment outside of the home.
- Having lost their mother before age 11 years.

f) F40—F49 Neurotic, Stress-Related and Somatoform Disorders

F40 Phobic Anxiety Disorders

F40.0 Agoraphobia

Anxiety that is restricted to crowds, public places, travelling away from home and travelling alone, and the psychological or autonomic response must be a manifestation of anxiety, not a delusion or obsession, and avoidance of the phobic situation must be a prominent feature.

F40.1 Social Phobias

Anxiety that is restricted to social situations, centred around fear of scrutiny by other people either face to face or in small groups (not crowds), and the psychological or autonomic response must be a manifestation of anxiety, not a delusion or obsession, and the phobic situation is avoided where possible.

F40.2 Specific Phobias

Anxiety that is restricted to specific situations, for example, animals, heights, enclosed spaces, etc., and the psychological or autonomic response must be a manifestation of anxiety, not a delusion or obsession, and the phobic situation is avoided where possible.

F41 Other Anxiety Disorders

F41.0 Panic Disorder

Recurrent attacks of unpredictable panic, with autonomic features, not related to a phobia or a particular situation.

F41.1 Generalised Anxiety Disorder

Generalised and persistent anxiety, associated with motor restlessness and autonomic overactivity, unrelated to environmental circumstances, occurring most days, lasting at least several weeks.

F41.2 Mixed Anxiety and Depressive Disorder

When depression and anxiety are both present, but neither predominant to justify a separate diagnosis.

F42 Obsessive-Compulsive Disorder

Recurrent obsessional thoughts or compulsive acts on most days for at least two weeks, unsuccessfully resisted, unpleasantly repetitive, and recognised as the individual's own thoughts.

F43 Reaction to Severe Stress

F43.1 Post-Traumatic Stress Disorder

Within six months of a 'traumatic event of exceptional severity', repeated reliving of the trauma through 'flashbacks' or dreams; associated with hypervigilance and autonomic arousal.

F45 Somatoform Disorder

Physical symptoms where medical investigation hasn't found a cause and are thought to be due to psychiatric processes.

F45.0 Somatisation Disorder

Multiple, recurring, frequently changing physical symptoms, occurring for at least two years.
   Also referred to as Briquet disorder and multiple psychosomatic disorder.
   This is *not* malingering, where the patient consciously simulates an illness.
   This is *not* Munchausen syndrome, where the patient deliberately harms the body to receive medical attention.

F45.2 Hypochondriacal Disorder

Persistent preoccupation with having one or more particular disorders. Attention is usually focused upon only one or two body systems.

Somatisation: worry about non-specific symptoms	vs.	Hypochondriasis: worry about specific physical disorders

F45.3 Somatoform Autonomic Dysfunction

Collection of symptoms that suggest they are due to autonomic innervation.

F45.4 Persistent Somatoform Pain Disorder

Predominant complaint is of unmanageable pain, which cannot be explained by a physiological disorder.

It is associated with emotional conflict or psychosocial problems.

The presentation results in increased in support and attention.

DSM-IV includes:

Conversion disorder—a neurological complaint triggered by psychiatric stress, usually presenting as weakness, paralysis and pseudoseizures. 'La belle indifference' refers to the patient who isn't distressed by such sudden symptoms.

Body dysmorphic disorder—where there is an overvalued false idea that a body part, often the nose, digits or skin, is grossly defective.

g) F50—F59 Behavioural Syndromes Associated With Physiological Disturbances and Physical Factors

F50 Eating Disorders

F50.0 Anorexia Nervosa (AN)

Characterised by deliberate weight loss, induced and sustained.

BMI <17.5 or weight <85% of expected.

Distorted body image and intrusive overvalued idea regarding dread of fatness.

Usually presents with undernutrition with secondary endocrine and metabolic changes.

F50.1 Atypical Anorexia Nervosa (AN)

Fulfils some features of AN but clinical picture does not justify diagnosis, for example, amenorrhoea or fear of fatness may be absent in the presence of marked weight loss and weight-reducing behaviour.

F50.2 Bulimia Nervosa (BN)

Characterised by preoccupation with the control of body weight, leading to binge eating then purgative behaviour.

F50.3 Atypical Bulimia Nervosa

Fulfils some features of BN, but clinical picture does not justify that diagnosis, for example, recurrent bouts of overeating and use of purgatives without significant weight change.

Text Box 18.5

SCOFF Questions

Eating disorder can be screened for using the SCOFF questions:
Do you every deliberately make yourself sick?
Do you ever worry you've lost control of the amount you eat?
Have you ever lost more than one stone in three months?
Do you believe you are fat when others say you are too thin?
Does food dominate your thoughts and life?
Scoring of two or more indicates likely AN or BN.

---

h) F60—F69 Disorders of Adult Personality and Behaviour

Screening tools for personality disorders:

The Standardisation of Assessment of Personality Abbreviated Scale (SAPAS) uses clinician interview for eight Yes/No questions attracting 1 score each; scoring >3 warrants further assessment.

The International Personality Disorder Examination screen (IPDE) uses a semi-structured interview and a questionnaire that corresponds to ICD-10 and DSM-IV.

The Iowa Personality Disorder Screen (IPDS) uses interview to assess 11 criteria.

In DSM-IV, schizoptypy is classified under schizotypal personality disorder, but in ICD-10 it is coded with schizophrenia as schizotypal disorder.

DSM-IV codes personality disorders into clusters:

Cluster A—paranoid, schizoid and schizotypal personality disorder.
Cluster B—narcissistic, borderline, antisocial and histrionic personality disorder.
Cluster C—obsessive compulsive, dependent and avoidant personality disorder.

Notes

1. Kaplan, H. I, and B. J. Sadock. (2007). *Concise Textbook of Clinical Psychiatry.* Philadelphia, PA: Lippincott Williams & Wilkins.
2. Kaplan HI, Sadock BJ. (2007) *Concise Textbook of Clinical Psychiatry.* Philadelphia, PA: Lippincott Williams & Wilkins.
3. Tandon R. (2014). Schizophrenia and Other Psychotic Disorders in Diagnostic and Statistical Manual of Mental Disorders (DSM)-5: Clinical Implications of Revisions from DSM-IV. *Indian Journal of Psychological Medicine*, 36 (3), 223–225.
4. Leff, J., N. Sartorius, A. Jablensky, A. Korten, and G. Ernberg. The International Pilot Study of Schizophrenia: Five-Year Follow-Up Findings. *Psychological Medicine*, 22 (1): 131–145.

5. Kuhn, R., and C. H. Cahn. (2004). Eugen Bleuler's Concepts of Psychopathology. *History of Psychiatry* 15 (59 Pt 3): 361–366.
6. Leff, J., and C. Vaughn. (1985). *Expressed Emotion in Families*. New York: Guilford Press.
7. Brown, G. W., and T. O. Harris. (1978). *Social Origins of Depression: A Study of Psychiatric Disorder in Women*. London: Tavistock.

Index

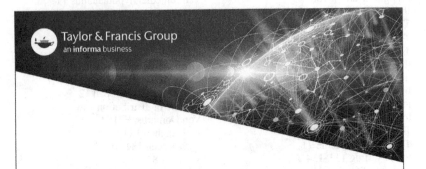

Printed in the United States
by Baker & Taylor Publisher Services